The Ultimate Career Guide

for medical students and foundation doctors

The Ultimate Career Guide

for medical students and foundation doctors

Samuel Latham MBChB MBA

and

Amelle Ra MBChB LLM

Scion

© **Scion Publishing Ltd, 2021**
First published 2021

All rights reserved. No part of this book may be reproduced or transmitted, in any form or by any means, without permission.

A CIP catalogue record for this book is available from the British Library.

ISBN 9781911510833

Scion Publishing Limited
The Old Hayloft, Vantage Business Park, Bloxham Road, Banbury OX16 9UX, UK

www.scionpublishing.com

Important Note from the Publisher
The information contained within this book was obtained by Scion Publishing Ltd from sources believed by us to be reliable. However, while every effort has been made to ensure its accuracy, no responsibility for loss or injury whatsoever occasioned to any person acting or refraining from action as a result of information contained herein can be accepted by the authors or publishers.

Readers are reminded that medicine is a constantly evolving science and while the authors and publishers have ensured that all dosages, applications and practices are based on current indications, there may be specific practices which differ between communities. You should always follow the guidelines laid down by the manufacturers of specific products and the relevant authorities in the country in which you are practising.

Although every effort has been made to ensure that all owners of copyright material have been acknowledged in this publication, we would be pleased to acknowledge in subsequent reprints or editions any omissions brought to our attention.

Registered names, trademarks, etc. used in this book, even when not marked as such, are not to be considered unprotected by law.

Cover design by Andrew Magee Design
Typeset by Medlar Publishing Solutions Pvt Ltd, India
Printed in the UK

Last digit is the print number: 10 9 8 7 6 5 4 3 2 1

Contents

Preface ix

Acknowledgements xi

Abbreviations xiii

CHAPTER 1
Essential principles 1

CHAPTER 2
Aspects of a successful CV 5
2.1 Example CV 7

CHAPTER 3
Medical portfolios 11

CHAPTER 4
The experts 13

CHAPTER 5
Academic success 15
5.1 Degrees and qualifications 15
5.2 Examinations 17
5.3 Research 19
5.4 How points are allocated for academic success 25
5.5 Top tips for medical students 33
5.6 Advice from the experts 34

CHAPTER 6
Prizes and awards 37
6.1 Presentation competitions 38
6.2 Essay competitions 38

6.3	Bursaries, scholarships and grants	39
6.4	Medical school prizes	40
6.5	NHS awards	41
6.6	Miscellaneous	42
6.7	How points are allocated for prizes and awards	42
6.8	Top tips for medical students	44
6.9	Advice from the experts	44

CHAPTER 7
Leadership and management 47

7.1	Committee member	47
7.2	Representative	48
7.3	Founder	48
7.4	Fellow and scholar	52
7.5	Non-healthcare related roles	53
7.6	How points are allocated for leadership and management	53
7.7	Top tips for medical students	54
7.8	Advice from the experts	55

CHAPTER 8
Teaching others 57

8.1	Contributing to teaching	57
8.2	Designing a teaching programme	58
8.3	Teaching qualifications	59
8.4	How points are allocated for teaching others	60
8.5	Top tips for medical students	64
8.6	Advice from the experts	65

CHAPTER 9
Quality improvement 67

9.1	How points are allocated for quality improvement	69
9.2	Top tips for medical students	71
9.3	Advice from the experts	71

CHAPTER 10
Demonstrating commitment 73

10.1	Ways to demonstrate commitment	73
10.2	How points are allocated for demonstrating commitment	78
10.3	Top tips for medical students	79
10.4	Advice from the experts	79

CHAPTER 11
General tips for building your portfolio 81

CHAPTER 12
The foundation programme (FY1 and FY2). 83

12.1 Standard UK foundation programme. 83
12.2 Academic foundation programme 91
12.3 Foundation priority programme 93
12.4 Psychiatry foundation fellowship programme 93
12.5 Top tips for medical students 95

CHAPTER 13
Taking a FY3 97

13.1 FY3 clinical roles 97
13.2 FY3 logistics 100
13.3 FY3 pitfalls 102
13.4 Top tips for medical students 103
13.5 Advice from the experts 104

CHAPTER 14
NHS training routes 107

14.1 Core (internal) medicine training and higher
     specialty training 107
14.2 Core surgical training and higher specialty training. 109
14.3 Run-through training programmes 109
14.4 Acute care common stem 113
14.5 Competition ratios 113
14.6 Academic training routes. 117
14.7 Top tips for medical students 118

CHAPTER 15
General practice. 119

15.1 Multi-Specialty Recruitment Assessment 119
15.2 Selection centre face-to-face assessment 121
15.3 GP specialty training 121
15.4 Portfolio GP 122
15.5 Insight from GPs and GP trainees 123

CHAPTER 16
Alternative careers 127

16.1   Military doctor 127
16.2   Entrepreneurship 132
16.3   Pharmaceutical physician 136
16.4   Management consulting 140
16.5   Medico-legal careers 143
16.6   Top tips for medical students 148

CHAPTER 17
Working abroad 149

17.1   The USA 149
17.2   Canada 150
17.3   Australia 151
17.4   New Zealand 153
17.5   Points to consider about working abroad 154
17.6   Top tips for medical students 156

CHAPTER 18
Not having a career goal 157

18.1 Top tips for medical students 159
18.2 Advice from the experts 159

CHAPTER 19
Staying out of trouble 163

Preface

This guide is designed to enhance the employability of prospective and current doctors. Whether you are a sixth-form student who has just received an offer to study medicine, or whether you're a junior doctor looking to take the next step towards your chosen specialty, this guide can be used to help you achieve your career goals. The material in this guide has been created with help from doctors who have tasted both success and failure. These doctors have worked within different specialties and NHS Trusts. They have also experienced careers outside of medicine and overseas. Whichever career path you want to take, and even if you want to work abroad, the information in this guide will be relevant to you and it will give you a head start against the competition. It may also help you decide which career path to take!

Graduating from medical school and becoming a doctor does not guarantee you a jaw-dropping career. In order to progress, there are certain boxes you need to tick and certain traits you need to possess. These are not signposted often enough throughout medical school and you risk missing opportunities to pursue them if not aware of their significance. Unfortunately, as the first person in my family to attend medical school, I missed many of these opportunities. After graduation, I was swiftly propelled into the NHS and began work as a FY1. I wanted to teach medical students at my Trust and provide them with the most valuable information I could offer. To do this, I created a teaching programme, titled 'What They Don't Teach You at Medical School'. It was clear that medical students receive enough teaching on becoming doctors, but do not receive enough on having happy and successful careers. This lecture series earned overwhelmingly positive feedback. Students would stay behind to ask questions, request copies of the slides, and they would commonly ask me to add more lectures to the series. Over time the material grew and evolved. Eventually, it became clear to me – the best way for me to deliver the content was through a written guide.

That is when I sought collaboration with Dr Amelle Ra. Her knowledge, determination, attention to detail, and network have proven to be immeasurable assets for the creation of this guide. The written content of the book is the product of our equal contributions as co-authors.

Samuel Latham

Acknowledgements

Samuel Latham

Thank you to my family for all of their hard work and encouragement. Particularly my grandparents Joan, Charlie, Marian and Bob, my parents Claire and Phil, and my brothers Phil and Lewis. This guide is a by-product of their consistent support. In addition, the contributions made by talented doctors throughout this guide offer immeasurable value to readers. I feel privileged to have met these doctors and I am very thankful for their inspiring words.

Amelle Ra

I would like to thank my loving family and friends for their ongoing help and support. Special thanks must go to my grandparents, parents, Neil, my uncles and my sister Erin. Without their continuous encouragement, this guide would not have been possible and I would not be the person I am today. I am also very grateful for the contributions made by exemplary doctors throughout. Thanks to them, readers of this book will be better equipped to pursue their own unique and rewarding careers.

Thank you all

Abbreviations

ACCS	acute care common stem
ACF	Academic Clinical Fellowship
AFP	Academic Foundation Programme
ARCP	annual review of competence progression
CST	core surgical training
ECFMG	Educational Commission for Foreign Medical Graduates
EPM	educational performance measure
FMLM	Faculty of Medical Leadership and Management
FPAS	Foundation Programme Application System
FPCC	Foundation Programme Certificate of Completion
FPP	Foundation Priority Programme
FY	foundation year
GDMO	general duties medical officer
IMG	international medical graduate
IMT	internal medicine training
MSRA	Multi-Specialty Recruitment Assessment
OOPE	out of programme for clinical experience
OOPT	out of programme for approved clinical training
OSCE	objective structured clinical exam
PACEs	practical assessment of clinical examination skills
PDSA	plan, do, study, act
PFF	Psychiatry Foundation Fellowship
PMST	pharmaceutical medicine specialty training
PQO	Professionally Qualified Officer
SJT	situational judgement test
STS	single transferable score
USMLE	United States Medical Licensing Examination

CHAPTER 1

Essential principles

We believe that there are seven key principles that will facilitate your journey towards your ideal career. We do not expect you to think about these principles every day. However, they are common themes throughout this guide. We will reinforce their value to you by using quick reminders. This reinforcement will help you adopt these principles into your everyday life and thus help you to unlock your true potential.

- **Don't ask, don't get**

In medicine, as in life, people you meet will not prioritise your future. Very often, you will come across people that are willing to help you but will not do so without prompting. That is why it is so important to ask for the things that you want. Never feel like you are being too cheeky. If being direct is not your style, there are other ways around this. Which leads us nicely onto the second principle.

- **Learn to influence others**

The ability to make people want to help you is invaluable. The fact that you are a doctor, or about to become one, means that you are probably a decent person (deep down). Try to show your friendly and grateful side as much as possible. Learning how to ask for favours in a polite way is also indispensable. Never underestimate the value of a beautifully constructed email!

- **Always have a plan**

Those who fail to make a plan, plan to fail. Creating short-term and long-term objectives is essential to motivating yourself and monitoring your progress. The plan does not have to be masterful, it just needs to be enough to get you out of bed on weekends; for example, planning to start revision on a specific date. A very good way of making plans is to create a to-do list.

- **You can never be too organised**

There are few things more frustrating than when you miss an opportunity due to being disorganised. One way you can avoid this is by using the calendar on your phone. Another way is by digitally backing up all of your important documents and storing them neatly in folders. Being organised helps you work efficiently and shows others that you are reliable.

- **Diversify or die**

The key to this principle is not restricting your assets. Those who have only one expertise are at risk of becoming irrelevant. When given the opportunity to diversify your skillset or knowledge base, grab it with both hands. Examples of this include formal qualifications, internships, taster weeks, and joining clubs or societies.

- **Fake it until you make it**

When you do not feel quite ready to commit to an opportunity, remember that learning on the job is the quickest way to learn. Try not to let fear of failure stand in your way. Time is never wasted when you are active. Sometimes, just having the confidence to give it your best shot is enough to seize an opportunity.

- **Avoid burnout**

Do not let work take over your life. As a doctor, burnout is something you have to take great care to avoid. It is so important to have a healthy lifestyle and to regularly free your mind from work. Arrange activities with your friends and try to explore new places. Completely escaping your responsibilities will allow you to recharge and work much more effectively in the long run.

In addition to the use of the seven key principles, you will see that throughout the book we have assigned you with homework. We strongly advise you to engage with this. Only truly valuable tasks have been selected as homework and many of them can be completed effortlessly.

ESSENTIAL PRINCIPLES · CHAPTER 1

> **HOMEWORK 1:**
> Make a to-do list and keep it updated, begin to use the calendar on your phone, arrange the files on your laptop, organise a fun activity with friends to look forward to.

CHAPTER 2

Aspects of a successful CV

Medicine is a fantastic, unique career with endless possibilities. However, just like in any other career, you will need a strong CV to stand a chance of being accepted for your dream job. Applying for a job in medicine is a competitive process and, unfortunately for doctors, other doctors provide stiff competition. To rub salt into the wound, the more sought-after your dream job is, the fiercer the competition will be. With this in mind, your focus may instinctively drift towards achieving the best grades at medical school and this is, of course, important. Nevertheless, you will have a more successful career by choosing to prioritise the development of your CV (providing that you still pass all of your exams) and we will explain the rationale for this later in this chapter.

Often, you will hear medics refer to their portfolio rather than to their CV. In simple terms, they are referring to the same thing. The most significant difference is that a portfolio also contains evidence to validate your claims, e.g. certificates and feedback forms. It will therefore be substantially larger than your CV. When applying for specialty positions, recruiters will score your portfolio in terms of content and layout and this score will be used to determine if you are suitable for interview. It is therefore crucial for doctors to construct a strong CV, which can also become part of their portfolio.

First, it is important that your CV is always tailored to the role for which you are applying. You may find yourself applying for varying roles simultaneously and so it is useful to create a 'master CV' that contains all of your experience, and which can then be trimmed and adjusted accordingly. Furthermore, you should always try to pre-empt the recruiter's needs and preferences. It is becoming increasingly important for applicants to show competency in handling data and operating technology. Bear this in mind when you are applying for a role and attempt to fulfil all of the likely criteria. Using the same logic, it is crucial to update your CV as new trends and advances enter the field of play.

In the box below, we have provided you with a number of potential headings for your master CV. For each heading we have given descriptions of information you might want to include. Feel free to adjust or merge these when creating headings for your own CV. You will find that a lot of the information you want to include could be applied to multiple headings. For example, a prize won at medical school could fall under the 'Education' heading or the 'Achievements' heading. Similarly, being a committee member of a charity may be considered as 'Leadership' or 'Volunteering' experience. It is up to you to structure your CV so that it flows nicely and doesn't repeat itself.

> **Personal information:** full name (plus titles and degrees), city in which you live, email address, telephone number, social media handles.
>
> **Mission statement:** a short summary of your strengths, values, and what you hope to achieve in your career.
>
> **Professional experience:** job titles and responsibilities, your knowledge/skills development, and significant landmarks you have reached.
>
> **Education:** GCSE and A-level qualifications, degrees, diplomas.
>
> **Research experience:** publications, presentations.
>
> **Teaching:** sessions/programmes you have developed or delivered, creation of educational literature, and participation in formal teaching/training.
>
> **Leadership:** formal roles and responsibilities, your knowledge/skills development, and significant landmarks you have reached.
>
> **Achievements:** prizes, awards, scholarships, bursaries.
>
> **Volunteering:** charitable efforts.
>
> **Additional skills:** languages, IT proficiencies, further relevant qualifications.
>
> **Interests:** activities in your spare time that depict your character.

ASPECTS OF A SUCCESSFUL CV — CHAPTER 2

Things to remember:

- Display text beneath each heading in chronological order and provide a transparent timeline (year of starting and year of finishing).
- Bullet points can be space efficient and punchy.
- Widen the margins on your paper, use 1.15 spacing, font size 10–12 and select a font that is clear and formal.
- Confine your CV to 2 pages of A4 paper when sending it to an employer. When creating a master CV, try to restrict it to 3 or 4 pages.
- Remember that you are allowed to be creative. A CV is just a piece of paper that tells your story. There is nothing preventing you from including links to videos or showing off your graphic design abilities.

2.1 Example CV

Miss Denisha Smith MBChB BSc
denisha.smith@nhs.net | @dr_smith | 07987123654 | London

Denisha is a FY1 doctor with a demonstrated interest in otolaryngology. Her career goal is to become a consultant otolaryngologist and perform challenging surgeries. She is a talented scientist, team player, and conscientious worker. Her passions include research and charity work.

Professional experience

FY1 Doctor – Ashford and St Peter's Hospitals NHS Foundation Trust, Surrey (2021–present)
- Rotations: General Surgery, General Medicine, and Psychiatry
- Activities: Provided regular surgical-themed teaching sessions to final year medical students
- Taster week: Department of Otolaryngology, King's College Hospital NHS Foundation Trust

Medical Elective – Mnazi Mmoja, Zanzibar (2020)
- Contributed to patient care in surgery, internal medicine, paediatrics and gynaecology
- Gained exposure to tropical medicine

Shop Assistant – The Body Shop (2015–2020)
- Developed skills in sales and customer service

Education

Bachelor of Medicine, Bachelor of Surgery (MBChB) – University of Bristol (2015–2021)
- Winner of the best performance in summative OSCE prize
- Bristol Medical School Women's Rugby Football Club committee member

Applied Anatomy (BSc) – University of Bristol (2020)
- Enhanced my understanding of the principles of comparative anatomy
- Dissertation entitled 'Head and neck anatomy of mammals'

Catford High School (2001–2015)
- Honorary scholarship for consistently achieving high examination results
- A-level: AAA – Biology, Maths, Chemistry. GCSE: 5-A*, 5-A

Research experience

'The Future of Medical Education' (Commentary) – *Medical Education Journal* **(2020)**
- First author of this published article about futuristic teaching methods

'Bristol Medical School curriculum flaws and necessary changes: a survey-based study' (Oral Presentation) – London Research Society's Annual Conference (2019)
- Delivered an oral presentation regarding the results of a survey-based study, which identified the least favourable aspects of the Bristol Medical School curriculum and popular adjustments to improve them. Awarded 2nd place in the oral presentation competition.

Teaching

Surgical Masterclass Teaching – Bristol University Surgical Society (2020)
- Provided a comprehensive teaching session to thirty-five 3rd year medical students

- This session covered all surgical pathologies likely to appear in 3rd year summative assessments
- Collected formal feedback and identified areas for improving future sessions

OSCEs Examiner – Bristol Medical School (2020)
- Improved my ability to assess clinical performance and provide constructive feedback

Leadership

Vice-president – University of Bristol Otolaryngology Society (2019)
- Arranged teaching sessions for medical students and raised money for hearing loss charities

Achievements

Katherine Branson Essay Prize Winner – Medical Women's Federation (2019)
- Awarded for my essay entitled 'Women in Medicine – past, present, and future'

Commendation Prize for Science – Catford High School (2015)
- Awarded for my project related to sustainable energy

Gold Duke of Edinburgh's Award (2015)
- Completed all sections of this award programme, including: volunteering, physical activity, skills activity, expedition, and residential activity

Volunteering

Events First Aider – St John Ambulance (2013–2015)
- Developed first aid skills and provided care for my local community

Additional skills

Fluent in speaking French and proficient in Microsoft Office

Interests

Jazz music, environmentalism, women's rights, animal rights

📁 You can never be too organised

HOMEWORK 2:

Have a go at creating your master CV and keeping it updated. You may need to send your CV to hospitals when applying for medical electives. When rushed, it is surprisingly easy to forget things that should be included!

CHAPTER 3

Medical portfolios

As mentioned in the previous chapter, doctors must transform their CV into a portfolio when applying for specialties after FY1 and FY2. Each portfolio is scored by recruiters and will determine if the candidate is suitable for interview. Broadly speaking, every candidate will be scored on six different aspects of their portfolio. These six scores will then be combined to produce an overall score. Often, recruiters will establish a cut-off point, meaning candidates must gain a certain number of points to qualify for an interview. If successful in reaching interview, the overall score from the candidate's portfolio will then be considered in combination with their interview performance. Usually, a candidate will receive a score for their interview performance, which will be added to the overall score for their portfolio. This provides the basis for achieving a job offer.

The six aspects of a doctor's portfolio are as follows:
1. **Academic success**
2. **Prizes and awards**
3. **Leadership and management**
4. **Teaching others**
5. **Quality improvement**
6. **Demonstrating commitment**

These six aspects are equally important in every specialty. One could even argue that they are equally important in every career. Year after year, competition intensifies for jobs and if a candidate chooses to neglect one of the six aspects, they will be reducing their likelihood of successful applications. That is why it is so important to focus on all six of the aspects, rather than the ones that seem most interesting.

In each of *Chapters 5–10*, we will be dissecting one of these aspects in detail. Our aim is to provide you with all the crucial information that will help you build a well-rounded master CV and achieve maximum points for your portfolio. If you already have a specialty in mind, use an online search engine to find a copy of the latest portfolio self-assessment scoring guide. If you are uncertain about the specialty you want to apply for, try searching for the Internal Medicine Training (IMT) and the Core Surgical Training (CST) portfolio-scoring guides. They will both give you an indication of how strong your portfolio is currently and what you should aim for in the future.

> **HOMEWORK 3:**
>
> Use your master CV to highlight areas that require improvement, begin to think of ways to improve your CV, create a LinkedIn account, search for people who have admirable jobs and see what experience they have (use this as inspiration).

CHAPTER 4

The experts

Each of the following six chapters (and some chapters thereafter) contain take-home messages from doctors who have demonstrated excellence in their fields. These doctors have been through the process of applying for specialty training positions and have managed to secure their dream jobs. A brief profile for each doctor is set out below.

Professor Chloe Orkin
MBBCh (Wits), FRCP (London), MSc Infectious Diseases London School of Hygiene & Tropical Medicine, University of London

- Professor of HIV Medicine, Queen Mary University of London and Consultant Physician, Barts Health NHS Trust
- Current Vice President of Medical Women's Federation
- Immediate Past Chair of the British HIV Association
- Governing Council for International AIDS Society
- BME Lead for COVID (NIHR North Thames)

Dr Elaine Winkley
MBBS, FRCA

- Consultant Anaesthetist and Acute Pain Lead, Northumbria NHS Foundation Trust
- Clinical Lead for Sustainability in Healthcare, HEE North East and North Cumbria

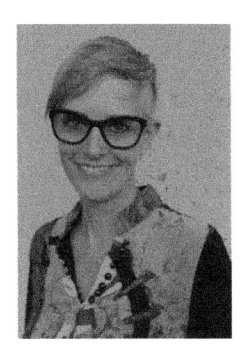

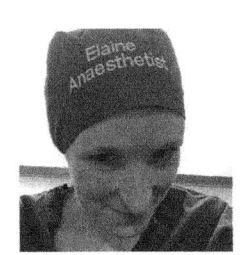

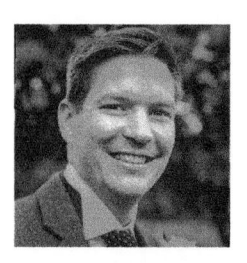

Mr Gareth Dobson
BSc (Hons), MBChB, MRCS, MRCS (ENT), ILM

- Neurosurgical Trainee (ST5 Neurosurgery)
- Former Core Surgical Trainee (ENT Themed)

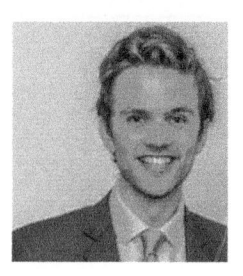

Dr George Miller
MBBS, BSc (Hons), MInstLM

- Public Health Registrar, Imperial College Healthcare NHS Trust
- Senior Director of The Healthcare Leadership Academy
- Former Academic Foundation Doctor, Guy's and St Thomas' NHS Foundation Trust

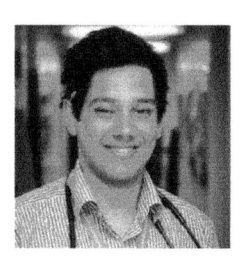

Dr Jeeves Wijesuriya
MBBS, MSc, AHEA

- GP Registrar ST3, Homerton University Hospital
- BMA UK Junior Doctors Committee Chair 2016–2019
- Trustee for Medical Aid Films Charity
- Care Quality Commission Special Advisor
- Former Academic Foundation Doctor

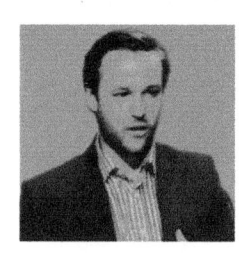

Dr Harrison Carter
BSc (Hons), MBChB (Bris), MPhil (Cantab), FRSA, FRSPH

- NHS England and NHS Improvement National Medical Director's Clinical Fellow
- Academic Foundation Doctor in Renal Medicine, Guy's and St Thomas' NHS Foundation Trust
- Former BMA UK Junior Doctors' Committee Executive, BMA UK Medical Students' Committee Chairman, and Member of BMA Council

CHAPTER 5

Academic success

In this chapter, we begin with very simple concepts and introduce you to the terminology that you must learn whilst at medical school. We will then go into greater detail and highlight ways for you to gain maximum points towards job applications. When it comes to academic success, there are endless opportunities, and to a large degree it does not really matter what subjects you decide to pursue. What does matter, is being able to complete processes successfully and being aware of how you can best evidence this. For the purposes of this book, academic success will be separated into three equally important criteria: degrees and qualifications, examinations, and research.

5.1 Degrees and qualifications

Graduating from medical school is an enormous achievement and will be one of the proudest moments of your life. If you are really bright and ambitious, then perhaps you can set yourself the goal of finishing in the top 10% of your year. If you achieve this, you will graduate with honours. Of course, this looks fantastic on your CV and will contribute points towards your job applications. If you are exceptionally bright and ambitious, and study medicine at a London university, why not aim for the Gold Medal prize? This is an annual competition whereby London medical schools nominate a small number of high achieving graduates to answer questions. With Sir Alexander Fleming amongst the list of previous winners, just participating in this competition will look fantastic on your CV.

If, like the majority of us, this all seems beyond reach, don't worry, you can still stand out from the crowd through hard work. One way of doing this is by completing another degree. Some readers may have completed an undergraduate degree before starting to study medicine. If this applies to you, then you are in luck. Completing an undergraduate degree before medicine will gain you points towards your job applications (even if that degree has nothing to do with medicine). The number of points gained will depend on the overall grade you achieved. If medicine is the first degree that you have studied, again do not worry, because there are plenty of opportunities for you to take time out of medicine and earn more degrees or qualifications.

'Intercalation' is a term that you will often hear. This represents an opportunity for medical students to take a year out of the medicine curriculum and to complete another degree during this time. Typically, the opportunity to 'intercalate' occurs after the 2nd, 3rd or 4th year of medicine (depending at which medical school you study). There are no restrictions with what degree you choose to study and where you decide to study it, as long as the course can be completed within one year. For example, you may consider studying a BSc in Anatomy (which is normally a three year course) because many universities offer a one year equivalent for intercalating medical students. In contrast, you may consider studying for a Master's degree in business or law. You may even wish to study abroad! Here is a list of degrees that are commonly chosen for intercalation:

Diversify or die

- Anatomy
- Biochemistry
- Bioethics
- Business
- Cancer biology
- Epidemiology
- Immunology
- Innovation
- Management

- Medical education
- Medical law
- Molecular biology
- Pharmacology
- Physiology
- Public health
- Surgery and anaesthesia
- Tropical medicine

It is also possible to be the first person to intercalate in a specific degree; all you need to do is contact the recruitment staff or course director to see if they are happy for you to complete the course within one year. You can also look for further information on **www.intercalate.co.uk**.

The number of points for intercalation that will contribute towards your job applications will depend on what type of degree you choose in addition to your overall grade. If you are worried about funding, there is a possibility to have your intercalation fully or partially funded by the NHS. Historically, medical students who intercalate are able to claim up to £9000 to fund their intercalation. This is because NHS England has agreed to fund university tuition fees for students who have already completed four years of an NHS degree. With the same logic in mind, this is why medical students in England do not have to pay tuition fees for their final year of university. Speak with your medical school faculty for further clarification of funding; funding options are different depending on which part of the UK you are from and often funding options are scarce for international students.

It is worth bearing in mind that completing an intercalated degree, or an undergraduate degree before medical school, are not the only ways to gain points in this category. Many doctors decide to take time out of their training to complete a postgraduate degree or diploma. Most commonly, doctors decide to do this after completing foundation years 1 and 2 (FY1 and FY2). However, there will be multiple opportunities to do this throughout your career.

> **HOMEWORK 4:**
>
> If it is almost time for you to decide whether or not you would like to intercalate, begin to research the potential options. If you have a particular university in mind, have a look at their online prospectus and see what courses can be completed within one year. If you would like to complete a specific degree, see if it is available at your current university, let the recruitment staff know you're interested and try to attend an open evening or lecture.

Always have a plan

5.2 Examinations

The thought of completing examinations that are not a part of your medical school curriculum might seem unnecessary. However, sitting extra exams is a great way of showing commitment to a specialty, gaining knowledge that will springboard your career, and earning extra points for your portfolio.

5.2.1 Medical student examinations

If you feel up to the challenge of completing an extra examination during medical school, then perhaps look into the Duke Elder Undergraduate Prize Examination. This exam is specifically for medical students and will gain you points towards ophthalmology applications. For more information, see ➔ **www.rcophth.ac.uk/examinations/duke-elder-undergraduate-prize-examination**.

5.2.2 Membership examinations

It is usually around FY1 or FY2 when doctors decide if they would like to pursue a career in 'core' medicine, 'core' surgery, acute care common stem (ACCS), or a 'run-through' specialty (see *Chapter 14* for clarification of these terms).

Applicants to 'core' medicine (also known as internal medicine training (IMT)) will benefit from completing the MRCP(UK) Part 1, which has a syllabus with a broad range of topics. Completion of this exam will not earn you points towards your initial job application, but it will provide evidence for your commitment to medicine and will provide you with additional knowledge that will be useful during interview. You need at least 12 months of experience in medical employment before sitting this exam. Data suggests that pass rates are highest when taken during FY2. Typically, alongside the commitment of working, doctors will revise for approximately 4 months before sitting this exam. There are then a further two parts of the MRCP(UK) to take: Part 2 written and Part 2 practical (practical assessment of clinical examination skills, or PACES). Passing all three parts is now mandatory before entering into higher specialist medical training in the UK. For more information, see ➔ **www.mrcpuk.org**.

Similarly, applicants of 'core' surgical training (CST) will benefit from completing Intercollegiate MRCS Part A. Unlike MRCP(UK) Part 1, completion of this exam will contribute points towards your portfolio by proving your commitment to surgery. Also, it is possible for FY1 doctors to sit this exam. Again, the syllabus includes a broad range of topics, and doctors typically spend about 4 months revising before the exam. There is a further part of Intercollegiate MRCS: Part B OSCE. Passing both parts is now mandatory before entering into higher specialist surgical training in the UK. For more information, see ➔ **www.rcseng.ac.uk/education-and-exams/exams**.

These exams are often referred to as 'membership exams' because their name stands for Membership of Royal College of Physicians/Surgeons. Examples of other membership (or sometimes 'fellowship', or even 'diplomate') exams that foundation doctors may consider completing or preparing for include:

- FRCEM primary (emergency medicine)
- FRCA primary (anaesthetics)
- MRCOG Part 1 (obstetrics and gynaecology)
- FRCOphth Part 1 (ophthalmology)
- MRCPCH theory examinations (paediatrics and child health)
- MRCPsych Paper A (psychiatry)
- DFPH (public health)
- FRCR Part 1 (radiology).

Note: *another exam to be aware of is the Multi-Specialty Recruitment Assessment (MSRA). This is a computer-based assessment which many specialties use to score candidates who apply for entry level training jobs. These specialties include general practice, obstetrics and gynaecology, psychiatry (Core and CAMHS), ophthalmology, radiology, community and sexual reproductive health, and neurosurgery. This exam is used as part of recruitment processes and so does not contribute to a doctor's portfolio (see Section 15.1 for more detail).*

HOMEWORK 5:

If you are reaching the end stages of medical school, consider whether you want to sit one of these exams during your foundation years. Then think about how you will rank your jobs for FY1 and FY2. A supernumerary rotation (without on-call commitments) around the time when you will start revision is definitely a good idea!

Always have a plan

5.3 Research

Arguably the biggest failure for medical students and doctors who wish to progress in their career is underestimating the value of research. NHS Trusts are constantly looking to pioneer advances in medical practice, and research is an indispensable part of this process because all advances must be proven by research before they are accepted. Recruiters for fiercely contested positions will therefore demand that candidates are able to evidence their participation in research. The most important concept to remember here is that it does not matter what your research is about, all that matters is proving your ability to conduct research effectively. For example, it is much more valuable for a plastic surgery candidate to have completed robust and meaningful research in the field of

psychiatry, than it is for them to have completed less robust and less meaningful research in the field of plastic surgery. Medical school provides the perfect opportunity to master the art of research. Here, we will cover the basics, including the different types of research, where to find research opportunities, publishing and presenting completed research, top research tips for medical students, and advice from the experts. Types of research studies are generally split into two categories:
- a primary research study is one that generates new data to be analysed
- a secondary research study collects and analyses data that already exists.

5.3.1 Types of primary research study

Primary research studies that you will become familiar with as part of your medical school curriculum include:
- Randomised controlled trial
- Cohort study
- Cross-sectional study
- Case–control study.

These study types are of high quality and are capable of producing impactful outcomes. However, as a medical student or foundation doctor, they are very difficult to become a part of. This is because they are expensive and time-consuming and require a lot of specialist knowledge and expertise. Generally, they are coordinated by researchers and consultants who are leading experts in their field. If an opportunity to become involved with one of these study types arises you should seize it, learn as much from the experience as possible, and seek further collaborations with the team in the future.

The types of primary research studies that medical students and foundation doctors are more likely to become a part of are:
- case reports – a description of a clinical case that reveals an interesting finding
- case series – when numerous cases are used.

These studies can be very thought-provoking and allow medical students and foundation doctors to evidence work that is highly specialised in a particular field. Unfortunately, clinical cases that are worthy of publication in a journal can be difficult to come across and finding them commonly requires help from senior doctors. Do not be afraid to ask consultants and registrars if they have any cases in mind that you could write up! For examples of case reports and guidance for authors, see ✓ www.casereports.bmj.com.

📢 Don't ask, don't get

5.3.2 Primary research studies and ethical approval

Ethical approval is needed for any research project that involves human participants, their tissue and/or data. This is to ensure that the participants of the research project are protected. Ethical approval is given by the Healthcare Research Authority (HRA) or by a research ethics committee; universities and NHS Trusts have their own committees. Normally, the consultant who is offering you the research opportunity will deal with this. However, you may need to speak to someone from the committee to ensure your project has ethical approval. This process ensures appropriate use of consent and anonymity. It can take a long time to submit your plans and to hear back from research ethics committees so do this as early as possible.

5.3.3 Types of secondary research studies

Like case reports and case series, secondary research study types are commonly carried out by medical students and foundation doctors. The most important examples can be found in *Table 5.1*.

Table 5.1: Types of secondary research study

Meta-analysis	This is a statistical method of combining the results of several studies that address a set of related research hypotheses. Almost all of the essential information from a meta-analysis can be displayed using a forest plot.
Systematic review	This is an in-depth summary of the published articles relevant to a defined research question. The articles are selected according to defined inclusion and exclusion criteria. The results within all of the selected articles are compared and an answer to the research question is evaluated.
Literature review	This is an article that reviews the key points of current knowledge in the scientific literature related to a particular topic. It should evaluate current understanding and identify unsolved questions. Rapid responses are a form of literature review that are considered for publication in journals. They are electronic letters to the editor that are related to published manuscripts.

Carrying out secondary research studies effectively is a skill that requires a lot of practice. Articles that address the research question might be difficult to track down and your work can quickly become out-dated by new studies. However, there is no need to generate new data, no need for ethical approval, and they can often be completed within a short timeframe. Medical students are commonly tasked with completing secondary research projects as part of their medical school curriculum. Apply yourself fully to this task and aim to produce a piece of work of which you are proud – it may be something you can later publish or present at a conference.

5.3.4 Clinical audit

Clinical audit is a process that looks to improve patient care and outcomes through a review of performance against set standards. Medical students and foundation doctors can easily become involved in clinical audits by asking consultants if there are any available. Usually, you will be tasked with data collection, which can involve trawling through documentation to find specific outcomes and entering those outcomes into a database (usually just a Microsoft Excel spreadsheet). Once complete, this data can be used to measure the quality of patient care and provide direction for improvements. Simply helping with data collection will not gain you any credit when it comes to job applications, but to ensure you gain credit, attempt to take ownership of the audit and present the findings at a departmental/regional/national meeting or conference. Even better, use the audit to write a research paper and aim to get it published. Clinical audits become much more significant if they inspire change and are repeated to confirm the change is actually beneficial. Once this happens, the clinical audit can be packaged as a quality improvement (QI) project (see *Chapter 9* for further details).

5.3.5 Miscellaneous

It is important to note that not all high-quality research projects fit into one of the categories mentioned above. For example, studies that focus on the results of a survey can uncover meaningful conclusions and can be published in journals and presented at conferences.

It is also possible to publish and present articles that are written about policy issues, ethics, education, personal views/commentaries, career issues, life as a medical student, etc. If this interests you, visit the websites of different journals to see what type of contributions they accept. A couple of great places to start are the *BMJ* and the *New England Journal of Medicine*:

- www.bmj.com/about-bmj/resources-authors/article-types
- www.nejm.org/author-center/article-types.

5.3.6 Publishing research

When the manuscript for your research project is complete you should submit it to a suitable journal. This is usually done via an online portal that can be found on the chosen journal's website; the consultant involved with the project will normally have some suitable journals in mind. The quality of a journal is generally shown by its impact factor, which is a score that quantifies the number of times a journal's articles are cited – in general, the higher the impact factor the better the quality of the journal. Make sure the journal is established enough to provide your work with a PubMed ID number once it has been published. If the journal is not established enough to provide this, you will miss out on points towards your future job applications.

After submission, the journal will either accept your work, potentially after asking you to make some minor amendments, or they will reject your work and give you feedback. Journals often have a maximum number of attempts for you to submit a paper for publication. Therefore, it is very important to be thorough before submitting your work. If your piece of work is accepted, congratulations! Try to obtain a copy of your work in the journal so you can include it in your portfolio. If your work is rejected, keep trying! There are plenty of journals out there. Although it has not worked out this time, the process of completing research and submitting it to a journal will stand you in great stead for the future.

5.3.7 Presenting research at a conference

At a conference, a research project can be presented orally or via a poster, perhaps as part of a conference presentation competition. Oral presentations involve standing in front of an audience and presenting your work (typically with the aid of a slideshow). Oral presentations last around 10–20 minutes before the floor is opened to questions. Poster presentations involve standing next to a poster that you have created, which depicts all of the crucial components of your research. Conference delegates will review your poster and may ask you to talk them through it. If your oral or poster presentation is a part of a competition, the audience will include a judging panel who will score your performance and decide if you are deserving of a prize. The aim is of course to win a prize (which looks great on your CV). If you do not win a prize, you will still gain a certificate for participating, which is often all you need to gain maximum points for the presentation section on your job applications. The process through which contestants are chosen to present their work usually involves submitting an abstract (a short summary of your research, usually with a maximum word count of around 300 words) online or via email. You will then select if you would like your application to be considered for an oral presentation, poster presentation, or both. There are a number of websites that list future conferences, such as:

- www.emedevents.com
- www.eventbrite.co.uk
- www.healthcareconferencesuk.co.uk
- www.conferenceseries.com
- www.medicsevents.co.uk

The more renowned the conference, the better that participating at it will appear on your CV. There are two main ways of determining the reputation of conferences:

1. Conferences that accept submissions from doctors and students are more highly regarded than conferences that only accept submissions from students.

2. International conferences are more highly regarded than national conferences, which are more highly regarded than regional conferences.

Top tips for winning oral and poster competitions:

- Know your topic well and be prepared to answer questions
- Microsoft PowerPoint is a useful tool for making slides for oral presentations and is arguably the best software for making posters

Fake it until you make it

ACADEMIC SUCCESS

- Do not overload slides and posters with text
- Try to make it as visual as possible
- Do not forget to include references
- Look online at prize-winning poster designs or slideshows and gain inspiration
- Practise presenting your work as much as you can before the big day!

5.3.8 Bursaries

You may encounter high costs associated with publishing articles and attending conferences. These costs can include open access charges for journal article submissions, and entrance fees, travel and accommodation for conferences. Medical schools often provide some form of funding to medical students who have their paper accepted by a journal or who are presenting their work at a conference. Speak with faculty to ensure you are not missing out on this. There are sometimes other sources of funding available, and it might also be worthwhile sending an email to the editor of the journal or the organisers of the conference to see if they have any recommendations. If you are a foundation doctor, you should ask journals for reduced charges and claim expenses for conferences as part of aspirational study leave.

5.4 How points are allocated for academic success

5.4.1 Degrees and qualifications

Tables 5.2–5.4 show the allocation of points for degrees and qualifications across training schemes for internal medicine and core surgery.

Table 5.2: Internal Medicine Training (IMT) 2021 – undergraduate degrees and qualifications

Option	Score
Degree obtained during medical course (e.g. intercalation, BSc, BA, etc.) – 1st class honours or equivalent	6
Degree obtained prior to starting medicine – 1st class honours or equivalent (can include non-medical degrees)	6
Degree obtained during medical course (e.g. intercalation, BSc, BA, etc.) – 2.1 or equivalent	3
Degree obtained prior to starting medicine – 2.1 or equivalent (can include non-medical degrees)	3

Reproduced from www.imtrecruitment.org.uk/recruitment-process/applying/application-scoring under the Open Government Licence v3.0.

Table 5.3: Internal Medicine Training (IMT) 2021 – postgraduate degrees and qualifications

Option	Score	Notes
PhD or DPhil – Doctor of Philosophy (can include non-medical qualifications)	6	If you undertook full-time research involving original work, usually of at least three years' duration, and ideally resulting in one or more peer-reviewed publication
MD – Doctor of Medicine, or MPhil – Master of Philosophy (can include non-medical qualifications)	5	The MD requires that you undertook full-time research involving original work, usually of at least two years' duration, and ideally resulting in one or more peer-reviewed publication
Master's level degree, e.g. MSc, MA, MRes, etc. (can include non-medical qualifications)	4	This must be a specific course that usually lasts for three university terms (or equivalent) and is 8 months or more duration (full-time equivalent); it must not be claimed for upgrading a bachelor's degree without further study as is offered in some universities
MD – Doctor of Medicine dissertation	3	If you undertook a dissertation (i.e. writing about a subject not using your own original research) with a relatively small amount of research content, and usually of 1 year or less in duration

(continued)

ACADEMIC SUCCESS CHAPTER 5

Table 5.3: *(continued)*

Option	Score	Notes
Other relevant postgraduate diploma or postgraduate certificate typically lasting between one and ten months (whole-time equivalent)	2	This option is for relevant postgraduate courses/modules – e.g. Diploma of Tropical Medicine and Hygiene; it is not permissible to claim points for partially completed qualifications, e.g. 1 year of a 3 year degree
		In addition to not being able to claim for the MRCP(UK) in this section, you also may not claim for other specialty membership examinations (e.g. MRCGP) or any similar qualifications from outside the UK (e.g. MRCP Ireland, FCPS Pakistan)
		Qualifications unrelated to medicine cannot be claimed for in this option

Reproduced from ✔ www.imtrecruitment.org.uk/recruitment-process/applying/application-scoring under the Open Government Licence v3.0.

Table 5.4: Core Surgical Training (CST) 2021 – degrees and qualifications

Option	Score	Notes
PhD or MD by additional research (level 8 qualifications); this can include non-medical qualifications	4	If you undertook full-time research involving original work, usually for a duration of at least 3 years, and ideally resulting in one or more peer-reviewed publication
Bachelor degree (level 6 qualification) in addition to primary medical qualification; 1st class honours or equivalent; this can include non-medical degrees or BDS	4	
Degree obtained during medical course (e.g. intercalation, BSc, BA, etc.) – 1st class honours or equivalent	3	This must be a specific course that usually lasts for three university terms (or equivalent) and is 8 months or more in duration (full time equivalent)
Taught and research Master's degrees (level 7 qualifications); this can include non-medical qualifications	3	If you undertook full-time research involving original work, usually for a duration of at least 2 years, and ideally resulting in one or more peer-reviewed publication

(continued)

Table 5.4: *(continued)*

Option	Score	Notes
Single-year postgraduate course (e.g. MSc, MA, MRes, etc.)	2	This must be a specific course that usually lasts for three university terms (or equivalent) and is 8 months or more in duration (full time equivalent); it must not be claimed for upgrading a bachelor's degree without further study as is offered in some universities
MPhil – Master of Philosophy	2	
Degree obtained during medical course (e.g. intercalation, BSc, BA, etc.) – 2.1 or equivalent	2	
Degree obtained prior to starting medicine – 2.1 or equivalent (can include non-medical degrees or BDS)	2	
Any other degrees or qualifications in addition to PMQ not covered in the above categories	1	For example: certificates or diplomas that do not fall into the above categories, partial higher degrees, intercalated degrees achieving 2.2 or lower
Primary medical qualification only	0	

Reproduced from the *2021 Core Surgical Training Self-Assessment Scoring Guidance for Candidates* handbook (available at ➤ https://coresurgeryinterview.com/resources/2021-Self-Assessment-Guidance-for-Candidates..pdf) under the Open Government Licence v3.0.

5.4.2 Additional exams

Table 5.5 shows the points awarded for the Duke Elder ophthalmology exam. Points gained for completing MRCS Part A can be found in *Section 10.2* as part of the demonstrating commitment chapter.

Table 5.5: Ophthalmology 2020 education scoring

Duke Elder scoring guide	Points
Finishing in the top 10% of entrants	2
Finishing in the top 60% of entrants	1

Adapted from ➤ www.severndeanery.nhs.uk/recruitment/vacancies/show/ophth-1-2020/portfolio-review-lib.

ACADEMIC SUCCESS　　　　　　　　　　　　　　　　　　　　　　　　　CHAPTER 5

5.4.3 Research

Tables 5.6–5.9 show the allocation of points for presentations and publications across training schemes for internal medicine and core surgery.

Table 5.6: Internal Medicine Training (IMT) 2021 – publications

Option	Score	Notes
I am first author, or joint first author, of two or more PubMed-cited original research publications (or in press)	8	For this option, you need to be first or joint first author in all of the publications to which you refer
I am co-author of two or more PubMed-cited original research publications (or in press)	7	This option can be interpreted as 'I am at least co-author in more than one...'
I am first author, or joint first author, of one PubMed-cited original research publication (or in press)	6	
I have written at least 50% of a book related to medicine (this does not include self-published books)	6	This refers to medicine in its broadest sense and not just hospital medicine; books must be published by an independent publishing house
I am co-author of one PubMed-cited original research publication (or in press)	5	
I am first author, joint first author, or co-author of more than one PubMed-cited other publication (or in press) such as editorials, reviews, case reports, letters, etc.	4	
I have written a chapter of a book related to medicine in its broadest sense (this does not include self-published books)	4	This refers to medicine in its broadest sense and not just hospital medicine; books must be published by an independent publishing house
I am first author, joint first author, or co-author of one PubMed-cited other publication (or in press) such as an editorial, review, case report, letter, etc.	3	
I have published one or more abstracts, non peer-reviewed articles or published articles that are not PubMed-cited	2	The article does not need to be medical in the strictest sense, but you must be able to justify its relevance to your application at any interview you attend

Reproduced from ➔ www.imtrecruitment.org.uk/recruitment-process/applying/application-scoring under the Open Government Licence v3.0.

Table 5.7: Internal Medicine Training (IMT) 2021 – presentations

Option	Score	Notes
An oral presentation, for which I was a first or second author, at a national or international medical meeting	8	National means that participation is routinely extended to, and accepted by, anyone in the country; as implied, international means participation extends beyond this
A poster, in which I was a first or second author, shown at a national or international medical meeting	5	National means that participation is routinely extended to, and accepted by, anyone in the country; as implied, international means participation extends beyond this
An oral presentation, in which I was a first or second author, given at a regional medical meeting	5	Regional means that participation is confined to, for example, a county, medical training region, health authority, or a recognised cluster of hospitals, extending beyond a city
An oral presentation, in which I was a first or second author, given at a local medical meeting	2	Local usually means participation is confined to a local hospital or university setting
A poster, in which I was a first or second author, shown at a regional or local medical meeting	2	As above

Reproduced from www.imtrecruitment.org.uk/recruitment-process/applying/application-scoring under the Open Government Licence v3.0.

Table 5.8: Core Surgical Training (CST) 2021 – publications

Options	Score	Notes
I am first author, or joint first author, of two or more PubMed-cited original research publications (or in press)	7	For this option, you need to be first or joint first author in all the publications to which you refer
I am co-author of two or more PubMed-cited original research publications (or in press)	6	This option can be interpreted as 'I am at least co-author in more than one...'
I am first author, or joint first author, of one PubMed-cited original research publication (or in press)	6	
I have written at least 50% of a book related to medicine (this does not include self-published books)	6	This refers to medicine in its broadest sense and not just hospital medicine; books must be published by an independent publishing house
I am co-author of one PubMed-cited original research publication (or in press)	4	
I am first author, joint first author, or co-author of more than one PubMed-cited other publication (or in press) such as editorials, reviews, case reports, letters, etc.	4	
I have written a chapter of a book related to medicine in its broadest sense (this does not include self-published books)	4	This refers to medicine in its broadest sense and not just hospital medicine; books must be published by an independent publishing house
I am first author, joint first author, or co-author of one PubMed-cited other publication (or in press) such as an editorial, review, case report, letter, etc.	2	

Reproduced from the *2021 Core Surgical Training Self-Assessment Scoring Guidance for Candidates* handbook (available at ➤ **https://coresurgeryinterview.com/resources/2021-Self-Assessment-Guidance-for-Candidates..pdf**) under the Open Government Licence v3.0.

Table 5.9: Core Surgical Training (CST) 2021 – presentations

Options	Score	Notes
I have given an oral presentation at a national or international medical meeting after being invited/selected to do so	6	
I have shown more than one poster at national or international medical meetings after being invited/selected to do so	5	
I have shown one poster at a national or international medical meeting after being invited/selected to do so	4	
I have given an oral presentation at a regional medical meeting after being invited/selected to do so	4	If you have contributed to a national or international oral presentation but did not give the presentation yourself, and have not used another option to claim this achievement, you may use this option
I have shown one or more posters at a regional medical meeting(s) after being invited/selected to do so	2	If you have contributed to a poster presented nationally or internationally, but were not first author, and have not used another option to claim this achievement, you may use this option
I have given an oral presentation, or shown one or more posters at a local medical meeting(s) after being invited/selected to do so	2	Regional and local meetings where you did not make the presentation or were only present for a poster question and answer session do not qualify

Reproduced from the *2021 Core Surgical Training Self-Assessment Scoring Guidance for Candidates* handbook (available at ➤ **https://coresurgeryinterview.com/resources/2021-Self-Assessment-Guidance-for-Candidates..pdf**) under the Open Government Licence v3.0.

> **Note:** When applying for a job, you may notice that more points are awarded for 'original' research than 'other' research. Original/other research is almost the same version of classification as primary/secondary research. Original research includes all types of primary research except case reports and case series, which (alongside literature reviews and letters) are classed as other research. Systematic reviews can be regarded as equivalent to an original research publication. Check the small print of the portfolio self-assessment guidance to be sure!

5.5 Top tips for medical students

- **Read up on potential degrees for intercalation.** Choosing to intercalate with a Master's rather than BSc often gains you more points for job applications and gives you better access to research. Make the most of your hard work and try to get your coursework and dissertation published and/or presented.

- **Do not worry about membership exams until your final year of medical school.** If you want to pursue a career in surgery, perhaps spend that summer revising for MRCS part 1 and sit the exam during FY1. That way you will capitalise on knowledge from finals remaining fresh in the memory. However, do not overwork yourself. The best way to revise is by signing up to an online question bank and going at a steady pace, e.g.
  ✔ www.pastest.com, ✔ https://www.emrcs.com,
  ✔ www.onexamination.com.

- **Identify the research opportunities to accept and the ones to turn down.** Don't be afraid to ask what the chances are of publication and conference acceptance. Do not do clinical audits for the sake of it (try to get the work published or presented).

- **Case reports can be a time-efficient way to gain points for research.**

- **Being competent at statistics is very useful** (pay attention during these lectures).

- **Collaborate wisely.** Recruiting colleagues who are able to contribute may be all that is needed to get the project over the finishing line.

- **Mention to supervisors and consultants that you are interested in research.** Follow this up with an email and explain the type of research you would like to become involved in, outline what you can bring to the table (e.g. good work ethic, free time, previous research experience, etc.), and tell them you would like to have the work published and presented.

- **You do not always have to rely on consultants**. There are usually registrars who will be able to help you. If you have an idea for a research project, write a plan for it and speak to a supervisor or mentor of yours for advice. Then crack on.

- **Freedom of information requests** are a great method of acquiring anonymous data from organisations.

5.6 Advice from the experts

Professor Chloe Orkin:

"Approach your consultants and ask for a research project. Be prepared to work out of hours to complete the work. Create fantastic slides – make friends with PowerPoint!"

Dr Elaine Winkley:

"Get involved early on. Search for opportunities online as well as in person."

Mr Gareth Dobson:

"Don't be afraid to say no. You will find a lot of offers to undertake projects will come your way. Some of these will be dead ends, with lots of time expenditure for little reward. If you do not think the project outcomes meet your needs, i.e. a publication or poster presentation, then avoid it."

Dr George Miller:

"Start with a letter to the editor of a journal so you can gain an understanding of how the publication process works. In other words, choose an article from a journal that interests you and provide the editor with a medical student's perspective on that article. Follow the journal's guidelines for authors and this will count as a publication once accepted."

Dr Jeeves Wijesuriya:

"The key with research and presentations is asking to get involved. Most senior academics work with or are associated with universities. The access you will have as students to these clinicians is virtually unparalleled. My advice would be to reach out to research staff, the Dean for research, or others, to see if there is anyone in need of help with their work. This is often a great way to get into research and also find a mentor who can help guide you through the world

of academia. My academic mentor was Sandra Nicholson who is now a professor of medical education and the lead for community based medical education. She has guided me throughout my academic career and been a tremendous colleague and friend to me. This doesn't always happen but being a little bit keen can go a long way, believe me!"

Dr Harrison Carter:

"No presentation is too small. For example, some will question the 'point' of having posters but the process of making an application – putting together a coherent abstract, seeking comments and writing a lay summary are useful and fundamental skills for a future academic career. In addition, my strong advice would be not just to apply to the conferences where work like yours is discussed. Think outside the box. Consider the softer skills that you may have gained whilst carrying out your research."

> **HOMEWORK 6:**
>
> Reach out to a consultant who you have been placed with. Email them and ask if there are any research opportunities for you to become involved with. Explain that you would like to be able to publish the work and present it at a conference.

- Learn to influence others
- Don't ask, don't get

CHAPTER 6

Prizes and awards

We all rely heavily on prizes and awards to determine quality. This is so ingrained in our behaviour that we probably fail to recognise the extent to which it happens. For example, in the history of athletics there are approximately 150 men who have run the 100 metres in less than 10 seconds and all of them were once capable of a very similar sprinting performance. However, it is mainly just the Olympic gold medal winners that are remembered. Another example can be seen when ordering a takeaway from one of two restaurants – the menus are very similar, as is the price and the customer feedback, but you notice that one of the restaurants has a TripAdvisor Certificate of Excellence whilst the other has not. In the majority of cases, this would become the deciding factor and you would probably select the restaurant with the certificate.

If we combine these two examples, the take home message is clear – prizes and awards have a powerful ability to make something more memorable and more desirable over a relatively long period of time. When it comes to recruitment, being more memorable and more desirable are two of the most important traits for candidates to possess. If we delve into it further, prizes and awards demonstrate determination and competitiveness, have the ability to completely transform the appearance of your CV, and are something you can refer to during an interview if the interviewer challenges the validity of your claims. Unquestionably, there is an element of luck when it comes to winning prizes and awards, but our advice is to keep trying until it happens. Persistence is key – to quote Gary Player (one of the most decorated golfers in history) "the harder I practise, the luckier I get".

In this chapter we will give you examples of different prizes and awards that you should try to obtain. We will illustrate the number of points you can gain for future job applications by winning prizes and awards. Lastly, we will give some of the important tactics to adopt when entering competitions.

6.1 Presentation competitions

As described in *Chapter 5*, prizes are often available for those who present research at conferences (see *Table 6.1*). It is noteworthy that if you win a prize at a national conference, this will count as winning a national prize.

Table 6.1: Presentation competitions

How to enter	Carry out research and submit an abstract to the conference organisers.
Pros	Even if you do not win, you will still get points towards your future job applications for presenting research at a conference.
Cons	If you are claiming points in the prizes and awards category of your portfolio for winning a presentation competition, you may not be able to also claim points for this in the presentation category. Therefore, you will have to win another prize/award or complete another presentation to gain maximum points.

6.2 Essay competitions

There are many Royal Societies, Royal Colleges, federations, and so on, which run essay competitions (*Table 6.2*). Details of these competitions can be found on their websites. Generally speaking, a title or topic will be released a month or so before the submission deadline. There is also a possibility that multiple essay writers will be given a prize or award.

Note: *If the competition is open to all students/doctors, this counts as a national prize.*

PRIZES AND AWARDS   CHAPTER 6

Table 6.2: Essay competitions

How to enter	Visit the websites of medical and surgical organisations. Examples include the Royal Colleges, Royal Societies, and federations. Check when they run their essay competitions and what the requirements are. A great place to start is the Royal Society of Medicine website: ➤ www.rsm.ac.uk/prizes-and-awards/prizes-for-students ➤ www.rsm.ac.uk/prizes-and-awards/prizes-for-trainees
Pros	The recommended word count for essays is usually significantly less than for a typical research paper. With regards to points for future job applications, it does not matter how renowned the organisation is, or of which branch of medicine the organisation is a part. If the essay is related to a specialty that you are interested in, the material may be something you are able to use in the future, i.e. for publication, presentation, or teaching sessions. Frequently, there is prize money awarded to the winner of these competitions.
Cons	Some recommended word counts are as large as research papers. Some essay competitions are hotly contested (you should try to target the more niche ones). It may be difficult to recycle the essay material into something useful for the future.

6.3 Bursaries, scholarships and grants

This involves receiving funding from an organisation (usually a university, Royal College, Royal Society or charity) to carry out a project. There is often a wide variety of project themes available. Bursaries, scholarships and grants (see *Table 6.3*) are normally awarded on a competitive basis and you will need to present your reasons for applying. You may be required to submit a written proposal, give an oral presentation, or attend an interview. Common examples of bursaries, scholarships and grants include funding to:
- carry out research
- go on a medical elective
- start a company
- complete a degree
- carry out voluntary work.

Table 6.3: Bursaries, scholarships and grants

How to enter	Visit the websites of organisations that are focused on medicine, surgery, charity and research. Examples include Royal Colleges, Royal Societies and registered charities. Check what options are available to enter and follow their recommendations. Here are some websites to get your search up and running: ➤ www.medschools.ac.uk/studying-medicine/medical-student-electives/elective-bursaries ➤ https://rmbf.org/medical-students/list-of-charitable-trusts ➤ www.rsm.ac.uk/prizes-and-awards/travel-grants-and-bursaries ➤ www.rcseng.ac.uk/standards-and-research/research/fellowships-awards-grants ➤ www.rcplondon.ac.uk/education-practice/funding-awards
Pros	They are capable of opening the door to many exciting opportunities, such as research projects and foreign travel.
Cons	They do not always gain you as many points as winning a national prize.

6.4 Medical school prizes

These are categorised by the percentage of students that they are awarded to. For you to gain points for job applications, the prize/distinction/merit must not be awarded to, for example, more than 20% of students on the course (and this must be evidenced). This percentage varies depending on the specialty you are applying to. There are many ways to win these awards that you will naturally encounter, such as performing well in exams and assignments. The classic example is receiving honours on your graduation day for finishing in the top 10% of the year. It is important to be aware that there are also medical school prizes that you must seek out to stand a chance of winning (see *Table 6.4*). Each medical school tends to host an end of year prize-giving evening. Prizes at these events are awarded for many things including essay competitions, extra-curricular projects, evidence of being an advocate of the medical school, evidence of an outstanding portfolio, evidence of leadership, etc. It is definitely worth tracking down the list of prizes that are available and setting your sights on more than one.

Table 6.4: Medical school prizes

How to enter	Confirm what prizes are available within your medical school and follow the recommendations.
Pros	Niche prizes at prize-giving evenings are less hotly contested and will gain you equally as many points for future job applications as the mainstream ones.
Cons	Finishing in the top 10% of the year requires a lot of hard work and astonishing ability. If performing well in exams is not your strong suit, claiming these points can be difficult.

6.5 NHS awards

There are awards up for grabs from a wide variety of regional NHS bodies, such as foundation schools, postgraduate deaneries, Trusts, hospitals, and primary care networks (see *Table 6.5*). There are also national prizes available from the NHS such as the parliamentary awards (✓ **www.england.nhs.uk/nhs-parliamentary-awards**).

NHS awards are typically given to staff only and so it might be difficult to obtain one whilst you are a medical student. Nevertheless, they are worth knowing about, because you will have the opportunity to win these before applying for specialty jobs.

Table 6.5: NHS awards

How to enter	Keep an eye out for emails and posters containing descriptions of awards. Search your Trust's website to find awards that might be available. Perhaps speak with the Foundation Programme Director at your Trust to see if they can provide any useful information.
Pros	There are lots of regional and local prizes to be won, you just need to be on the lookout.
Cons	Regional or local prizes do not gain you as many points as winning a national prize, which are unsurprisingly more difficult to win.

6.6 Miscellaneous

There are many prizes and awards that do not fit into any of the above classifications. For example, the Wellcome Trust has five prize categories for its annual photography competition. A theme related to healthcare is announced on the Wellcome Trust website and photos are judged according to their relevance and quality. The winner of each category receives £1250, and the overall winner receives a prize of £15,000. For more information see: ➤ https://wellcome.org/what-we-do/our-work/wellcome-photography-prize/2021.

6.7 How points are allocated for prizes and awards

Tables 6.6–6.7 show the points awarded for different awards and prizes across internal medicine and core surgical training.

Table 6.6: Internal Medicine Training (IMT) 2021 – Additional achievements

Option	Score	Notes
High-achievement award for primary medical qualification (e.g. honours or distinction); awarded to no more than the top 15%	6	If more than 15% of the year receive honours/distinction, etc., then it no longer marks you out as exceptional in this category
Awarded national prize related to medicine	4	This means that the prize is open to medical undergraduates and/or postgraduates in the country of training
One or more prizes/distinctions/merits related to parts of the medical course; awarded to no more than the top 20%	2	You may only claim this if you were in the top 20% of marks for part of the course on more than one occasion

Reproduced from ➤ www.imtrecruitment.org.uk/recruitment-process/applying/application-scoring under the Open Government Licence v3.0.

PRIZES AND AWARDS

Table 6.7: Core Surgical Training (CST) 2021 – Prizes/awards

Option	Score	Notes
Awarded national prize related to medicine	8	This means that the prize is open to medical undergraduates and/or postgraduates in the country of training
High-achievement award for primary medical qualification (e.g. honours or distinction); awarded to no more than the top 15%	6	If more than 15% of the year receive honours/distinction, etc., then it no longer marks you out as exceptional in this category
More than one prize/distinction/merit related to parts of the medical course or Foundation Programme; awarded to no more than the top 20%	4	You may only claim this if you were in the top 20% of marks for part of the course on more than one occasion
Awarded regional prize related to medicine	4	This means that the prize is open to medical undergraduates and/or medical postgraduates in the training region (e.g. foundation school or postgraduate deanery)
One prize/distinction/merit related to parts of the medical course or foundation training; awarded to no more than the top 20%	3	You may only claim this if you were in the top 20% of marks for one part of the course/training programme
Awarded local prize related to medicine	2	This means that the prize is open to medical undergraduates and/or medical postgraduates in a locality/organisation (e.g. NHS Trust, hospital, primary care network)
Scholarship/bursary/equivalent awarded during medical undergraduate training or foundation training	2	

Reproduced from the *2021 Core Surgical Training Self-Assessment Scoring Guidance for Candidates* handbook (available at ➤ https://coresurgeryinterview.com/resources/2021-Self-Assessment-Guidance-for-Candidates..pdf) under the Open Government Licence v3.0.

6.8 Top tips for medical students

- **Ensure that you claim all of the points that you are entitled to.** Make sure that "top 10%" or "top 15%" (or whatever is required) is detailed on any certificate/letter from your medical school as evidence of a distinction or merit.
- **Keep your certificates safe and back up a digital copy.**
- **Keep a copy of the award-winning work as well.**
- **Try to show commitment to what it is you are interested in.** This might not gain you extra points in this category but will contribute to interview performance.
- **Niche awards are less hotly contested** but may still gain you maximum points.
- **If at first you do not succeed, recycle your work and keep trying!**

6.9 Advice from the experts

Professor Chloe Orkin:

"Look out for essay prizes, research awards and APPLY! That is the first step."

Dr Elaine Winkley:

"Hard work pays off and will be recognised in due course."

Mr Gareth Dobson:

"You have to be in it to win it. Prizes and awards are generally hard to obtain, however, there are a lot of opportunities available where they are offered. Try your luck. If you don't succeed, then you will have probably obtained another CV-boosting poster or presentation."

Dr George Miller:

"Seek out national awards, often very few students submit an application. The Royal Society of Medicine awards page is a good place to start."

Dr Jeeves Wijesuriya:

"Most universities will have a number of prizes, some of which are essay-based or exam-based that you can both prepare for and apply to. It's well worth considering given it will only help with your revision! There are also loads of organisations who have prizes and awards for essays available to early career doctors and medical students. Whether it's awards for patient information leaflets you may have created, or prizes for essays like those at some Royal Colleges, it's worth browsing and seeing what you might be able to submit."

Dr Harrison Carter:

"Search for them yourself. Particularly awards that have a monetary value to further research. Look at a wide range of organisations and societies, including charitable bodies supporting patients with the conditions that you're interested in. Seek internal university funding. Ask the leading supervisors and medical educators in your field of interest. Discuss with more senior doctors in your desired specialty."

HOMEWORK 7:

Plan ahead, look at what prizes are available for you in the future and begin to prepare for them.

Always have a plan

CHAPTER 7

Leadership and management

The role of a doctor has changed greatly over the years and no doubt will continue to do so. There are now an enormous variety of essential healthcare workers that come together as one team. For example, the staff on a general medical ward in a hospital might include a matron, nurse in charge, staff nurse, healthcare assistant, physician associate, pharmacist, physiotherapist, occupational therapist, dietitian, specialist nurse (e.g. diabetes, stroke, palliative care, tissue viability, oncology, infection control, etc.), ward clerk, medical student, and so on. This list does not include any of the staff that help to run wards, clinics, and theatres from behind the scenes. As a doctor, you are responsible for the overall care of your patients. To ensure your patients receive a high quality of care, you must demonstrate leadership and management skills to coordinate the input of every multidisciplinary team member. This will be the case throughout your entire career. It is therefore paramount for doctors to show that they are capable of being effective leaders and managers before they can climb the ranks. This also applies to medical students who are considering a career outside of medicine.

In this chapter we will give you examples of different leadership and managerial roles you can apply for. We will also illustrate the number of points you can gain for future job applications by carrying out these roles.

7.1 Committee member

Becoming a committee member of an organisation is a simple process. First, you have to be a member of the organisation, which usually involves just signing up and perhaps paying a fee. Secondly, you should do some investigating to learn how the organisation is structured and how the committee is set up. It is always useful to speak to a committee member to find out this information and to gain an understanding of what being a committee member entails.

The duties of a committee member generally include carrying out the responsibilities of your specific role, attending meetings on a regular basis, engaging in debate, voting on proposals, providing members with reliable information, and being an advocate. Thirdly, you must determine when the selection process for the next committee is taking place and prepare your application. Depending on the committee you are applying for, the application process could involve writing a proposal, delivering a pitch, and possibly an interview. Last, but not least, you need to apply for the position you want and give it everything you have got. The most important quality to show is enthusiasm. Some of the committee positions that medical students and junior doctors commonly apply for can be found in Table 7.1. Remember, you may not need prior experience to be elected and you might be able to run for these positions as a pair.

Fake it until you make it

Table 7.1: Committee positions

Medical students	Junior doctors
• Medical student society • Student specialty society	• BMA LNC member • Junior doctors' mess president

If you are interested in becoming involved with the BMA, see: www.bma.org.uk/what-we-do/get-involved.

7.2 Representative

This is similar to being a committee member (committees are often composed of representatives). The main difference is that you are less likely to be involved in making decisions and will be more involved with simply promoting the activities of the organisation. You may still have to attend meetings, but you are more likely to work independently. The application process is fundamentally the same as applying for a committee position.

7.3 Founder

If you have an idea for an organisation, you could become the founder and director. The organisation does not need to be related to the provision of healthcare for you to gain points towards your future job applications. However, if it is related to healthcare, this will potentially gain you more points. The key element is originality.

Common examples of organisations that medical students create include student societies, charities, and start-up companies.

7.3.1 Student society

Applications to create student societies are submitted to the students' union or guild. It is good to develop a blueprint of the organisational structure and the activities you will run before beginning your application. Most universities require a president, secretary, and treasurer to be appointed for each society. You will need support from other students that wish to take part (usually 10 of them). Your application should include details about the sustainability of the society (e.g. elections for future committees) and how it intends to recruit members. Once your application has been accepted, you will gain access to university facilities and potentially some funding. Try to avoid paying for anything as a lot of university resources can be used for free. If you need money, fundraising options include grants from your university, membership fees, ticket sales for events, and sponsorship. When your time is up, ensure the society is left in good hands – the bigger and better the society becomes, the more credit you will gain from establishing it.

7.3.2 Start-up company

Ask yourself, what problem are you trying to fix with your start-up company? Then consider if you are willing to dedicate your time to solving this problem. If you are not passionate about the potential impact of your start-up, there is a high risk of losing interest and abandoning it. Think about who your customers are going to be. Are they willing and able to pay for your product? Also, how will you target them? Next, you must do your market research. Determine who your competitors are and what makes you different to them. Ask around and see if the people you trust think your start-up is a good idea – would they be happy to buy your product? Write out a business plan that includes all of these crucial elements: business overview (including name), operating plan, market analysis, products and services, sales and marketing, competitor analysis, management team, and financial plan.

Once you have finalised the business plan (and before you receive any income), you should register your company. If you are setting up a private limited company, you can do this online. The cost can be as little as £12 and the company is registered within 24 hours (*www.gov.uk/set-up-limited-company*). Then it is time to start developing your product and making yourself visible. Meet other entrepreneurs who have start-ups and learn from them – a great way of doing this is applying for the NHS Clinical Entrepreneur training programme (➤ **www.england.nhs.uk/aac/what-we-do/how-can-the-aac-help-me/clinical-entrepreneur-training-programme**). Important information to seek out includes methods of fundraising. Apply for as many grants as possible so that you can avoid spending your own money. Only partner with investors who are willing to add enthusiasm and expertise. Further important information to seek out is regarding partnerships for product development. Do not be afraid to partner with someone that brings something new to the table. For instance, if you have an app idea related to medicine, then you should focus on the medical aspect of the business and partner with an app developer who will take care of the coding aspect.

Soon your start-up will begin to take shape and you will have to consider all the paperwork that you might not have thought about when initially developing your idea, such as: contracts, data protection, business insurance, protecting your intellectual property, licences and permits, registering for VAT, etc.

7.3.3 Charity

Just like with creating a start-up company, you should be passionate about your charity's mission. Thorough planning is always advised and you should write out a business plan that includes: charity overview (including name and purpose for public benefit), operational plan, market analysis, products and services, sales and marketing, competitor analysis, management team (i.e. at least three trustees and potential committees), and financial plan. The simplest way to operate is as an unregistered unincorporated charity; for instance, a charitable trust. It is often advisable to start off this way until the charity is functionally established. With these types of organisations:

- Trustees are appointed and are legally responsible for the activities of the charity.

- It is good practice to write and sign a trust deed to show that your organisation is legally charitable (a model can be found on the Charity Commission website – ➤ **www.gov.uk/government/publications/setting-up-a-charity-model-governing-documents**)

- You do not have to register with the Charity Commission (as long as the charity's income is less than £5000 per year).

- The charity cannot legally have employees, enter into contracts, control investments in its own name, or hold land on its own behalf.
- The charity does not automatically qualify for charity tax benefits and Gift Aid.

Once the charity is up and running, you should consider if it is worthwhile becoming a registered charity. *Table 7.2* outlines some of the potential benefits and drawbacks.

Table 7.2: Becoming a registered charity

Benefits	Drawbacks
• Registered charities are more trusted and so more likely to receive large donations • The charity can automatically qualify for charity tax benefits and Gift Aid • There is no £5000 income limit • There is no personal liability for trustees once the charity becomes incorporated • The charity is able to have employees, enter contracts, control investments, hold land • The charity is more likely to stand the test of time • Being the founder of a registered charity appears better on your CV	• The paperwork is complicated and time-consuming • The charity must strictly abide by its constitution • Making changes to the constitution takes up time and effort • The charity must report to its governing body, i.e. Charity Commission/Companies House

If the pros outweigh the cons for you and your fellow trustees, you must then contemplate what type of organisation you would like to become. There are three main types:
- Charitable incorporated organisation (CIO)
- Community interest company (CIC)
- Company limited by guarantee (can be registered as a charitable company).

The most popular option for smaller charities is to become a CIO. This is because CIOs do not have to report to Companies House and so are easier and cheaper to run. Once you have chosen your structure, it is then time to create a governing document. This is essentially a constitution that your charity must abide by. There are model constitutions for you to follow on the Charity Commission website

(⏵ **www.gov.uk/government/organisations/charity-commission**). After that has been completed, you are ready to register your charity. This can be done via the UK Government website (⏵ **www.gov.uk/setting-up-charity/register-your-charity**). The paperwork is extensive and can be confusing for those who are unfamiliar with legal and financial terminology. Nevertheless, they can be completed without professional help. The charity commission is an underfunded organisation and there can be some delay in being allocated a case manager and receiving confirmation of a decision (this can take up to 7 weeks). Some important things to bear in mind when moving forward (regardless of what charity type you opt for):

- Always be transparent with your stakeholders.
- Choose your trustees wisely, because their approval is needed for every big decision.
- Do not let the process of becoming registered distract you from the charity's mission.

7.4 Fellow and scholar

There are educational programmes that provide medical students and doctors with an opportunity to improve their leadership and management skills, for example:

- Faculty of Medical Leadership and Management (FMLM) – The National Medical Director's Clinical Fellow Scheme (⏵ **www.fmlm.ac.uk/programme-services/individual-support/national-medical-directors-clinical-fellow-scheme**)
- NHS Leadership Academy – Edward Jenner programme open to students (⏵ **www.leadershipacademy.nhs.uk**)
- Healthcare Leadership Academy – Scholars programme open to medical students (⏵ **www.thehealthcareleadership.academy**).

The person specifications and the levels of commitment that are necessary to complete these programmes vary. Some programmes can be completed in your spare time, whereas others demand full-time attendance throughout the year. Entry is on a competitive basis and applicants should expect to submit a CV and a personal statement. You might also be asked to attend an interview. Broadly speaking, amongst all leadership programmes, the curriculum will cover similar topics. It is important to read up on these programmes and to select one that best suits your schedule and reasons for applying

LEADERSHIP AND MANAGEMENT

(e.g. points for job applications will vary). Speak with previous fellows/scholars to see what they have gained from taking part.

7.5 Non-healthcare related roles

If you are pursuing a career in healthcare, it is advisable to evidence leadership and management skills within a healthcare-related setting. However, you can still gain credit for carrying out leadership and management roles outside of healthcare. This can be related to anything as long as you are able to provide a letter that shows your appointment to the position, the time period you held the position for, and the positive impact you were able to have. It is also very important to specify if this was a national position or a regional position. Common examples include roles within charities, sports teams, politics, creative arts, etc.

> **Note:** *To claim points when applying for specialty jobs for any type of leadership or management role, you must have held this role since starting your first undergraduate degree and for a minimum of six months.*

7.6 How points are allocated for leadership and management

Tables 7.3 and *7.4* show the points awarded for leadership and management within internal medical and core surgical training.

Table 7.3: Internal Medicine Training (IMT) 2021 – Leadership and management

Option	Score	Notes
I hold/have held a national/regional leadership or managerial role for 6 or more months and can demonstrate a positive impact	6	Examples include: BMA national executive, trainee representative of a specialist society or college, or a nationally held leadership and management fellowship. Charity, Scouts/Guides, sports, creative arts at a national or regional level
I hold/have held a local leadership or managerial role for 6 or more months and can demonstrate a positive impact	3	Examples include a role within one hospital or medical school such as junior doctors' mess president or trainee representative on a hospital committee. Charity, Scouts/Guides, sports, creative arts at a local level

Reproduced from www.imtrecruitment.org.uk/recruitment-process/applying/application-scoring under the Open Government Licence v3.0.

Table 7.4: Core Surgical Training (CST) 2021 – Leadership and management

Option	Score	Notes
I hold/have held a national leadership or managerial role related to the provision of healthcare for 6 or more months and can demonstrate a positive impact	8	Examples include: BMA national executive, trainee representative of a specialist society or college, or a nationally held leadership and management fellowship
I hold/have held a national leadership or managerial role in a non-medical voluntary capacity for 6 or more months and can demonstrate a positive impact	8	Examples include: charity, Scouts/Guides, sports, creative arts at a national level
I hold/have held a regional leadership or managerial role related to the provision of healthcare for 6 or more months and can demonstrate a positive impact	6	Examples include a role covering more than one hospital or covering a postgraduate training region
I hold/have held a regional leadership or managerial role in a non-medical voluntary capacity for 6 or more months and can demonstrate a positive impact	6	Examples include: charity, Scouts/Guides, sports, creative arts at a regional level
I hold/have held a local leadership or managerial role in a non-medical voluntary capacity for 6 or more months and can demonstrate a positive impact	4	Examples include a role within one hospital or medical school such as junior doctors' mess president or trainee representative on a hospital committee
I hold/have held a local leadership or managerial role in a non-medical voluntary capacity for 6 or more months and can demonstrate a positive impact	4	Examples include: charity, Scouts/Guides, sports, creative arts at a local level

Reproduced from the *2021 Core Surgical Training Self-Assessment Scoring Guidance for Candidates* handbook (available at ➔ https://coresurgeryinterview.com/resources/2021-Self-Assessment-Guidance-for-Candidates..pdf) under the Open Government Licence v3.0.

7.7 Top tips for medical students

- **Do not be afraid to ask for a letter of confirmation** from someone more senior than you. Email them shortly after you have stepped down from the position and then you are more likely to get a response.

- **It is perfectly reasonable to write a draft letter for yourself** (which should include confirmation of your appointment to the position, the time period you held the position for, the positive impact you were able to have, whether the position was national or regional). Say to the person who will be signing it for you that you have done this to save them time. Ask them to sign it after they have made any changes that they feel are necessary.
- **Get involved in something you are actually interested in.**
- **Try to show commitment to your desired career path.**
- **Kill many birds with few stones.** Use your role to become involved in research or to organise teaching for medical students.

📣 Don't ask, don't get

7.8 Advice from the experts

Professor Chloe Orkin:

"Start small. Try to notice what your consultants and registrars are doing and try to shadow them. Ask what you can do to help in running the clinic or ward rounds smoothly. Then look out for leadership and management fellowships with external organisations like the Royal College of Physicians and the National Institute for Health Research."

Dr Elaine Winkley:

"Take on roles and work that you are passionate about. If you have an idea that you are committed to, keep going with it – it can take years before all the hard work pays off and you have to be committed, enthusiastic and believe in it."

Mr Gareth Dobson:

"Put yourself forwards. Not all leadership and management experience comes from courses. Whilst courses support your CV and tick boxes, there are lots of leadership and management opportunities available within each department, whether this is organising the rota, leading ward rounds or service development projects. Be proactive, get involved and more leadership and management prospects will come your way."

Dr George Miller:

"Get involved with university societies that already exist, but be comfortable going through the process of starting your own too. Consider applying for a BMA or INSPIRE representative role."

Dr Jeeves Wijesuriya:

"The key to leadership and management is getting involved. Whether that's in your students' union, clubs and societies, or junior doctors' forums, the key to leadership and management is experience. If you turn up there is so much experience to be gained, and some of the roles that have most shaped my development have been by turning up and putting myself forward for things. This can seem like the most intimidating thing in the world sometimes, but I promise you it is worthwhile. The BMA has a number of regional and local committees that also come with access to leadership training and experience of chairing meetings. The Junior Doctor Forums at each Trust are a wonderful way of getting experience of management in local Trusts. The FMLM also offer really great fellowship roles that you could take advantage of to get insights into different types of organisations and practice too. These sorts of roles are open to all trainees and will help develop your skills and leadership style."

Dr Harrison Carter:

"Local medical school committees, the BMA, and foundation doctor committees are all great starting points. Consider contacting the Guardian of Safe Working or the Chief Executive of your Trust to see what other options there might be."

HOMEWORK 8:

Attempt to identify a leadership position that is within your grasp. Although this may not be the position you put on your specialty job application, it will give you a better chance of entering into better-regarded positions. When applying for a leadership position, you will often be asked – what previous leadership experience do you have? That is why it is important to start now, gain experience, and begin climbing the ladder.

Always have a plan

CHAPTER 8

Teaching others

The proven ability to proficiently teach others is very attractive for recruiters. This is true in all industries. An employee who is able to teach and pass on knowledge to others provides a great prospect for improving standards of work. Teaching can also give organisations an additional opportunity for income and heightened status. Furthermore, the benefits of teaching are not restricted to organisations; teaching provides employees with improved job satisfaction and variety in their work schedules. The value of teaching is recognised more in the healthcare industry than almost any other. Right through your junior doctor career, you will be given regular teaching and must evidence your attendance at teaching in order to progress through training. A culture whereby junior doctors are willing and able to provide teaching for one another and to medical students is always encouraged by Trusts. This plays a significant role in how Trusts are expected to function. The more teaching that happens within a Trust, the better. For this reason, once hospitals have been recognised for their contributions to training, they are frequently referred to as university teaching hospitals. If you are hoping to pursue a successful career in medicine, you must prove that you are capable of providing useful teaching and, broadly speaking, there are three ways of achieving this:

1. you can contribute to an existing teaching programme
2. you can design a teaching programme and contribute to its delivery – this is better because it shows originality, problem solving, and initiative
3. you can gain teaching qualifications.

8.1 Contributing to teaching

There are many teaching programmes that you will have the opportunity to contribute towards. These will include revision days, small group teaching and clinical skills sessions run by your university,

Trust or by a specialty society. You may also come across a group of medical students or junior doctors who are running their own teaching programme that you could become involved with.

There is an opportunity to show commitment to a specialty by delivering teaching on a specific topic. However, there are also plenty of other ways to show commitment to a specialty. Overall, the topic that you are teaching does not matter much. We recommend signing up to teach a topic that you classically struggle with, because this will push you to learn more about it.

With all of the teaching sessions you carry out, you must ensure that the attendees fill out feedback forms – these can be completed in electronic or paper form (just remember to keep them somewhere safe once they have been filled out). You must also ask the person who is in charge of the programme to provide you with a signed letter. This letter must include information regarding how often you delivered the teaching and what time period this covered. To be on the safe side, we advise that teaching should be performed at least on a weekly basis for it to be considered as regular. Furthermore, the time period of this regular teaching should cover more than 3 months. A letter that confirms both of these elements will ensure that you are able to claim points for teaching on your future job applications.

8.2 Designing a teaching programme

Perhaps the easiest way to do this whilst you are a medical student is by working alongside a specialty society. If the society is registered with the students' union or guild, it will have access to university facilities and will be more likely to attract attendees to its events. There is potential to design a teaching programme through collaboration with your medical school or Trust and for this to become a part of the curriculum. However, this will take a lot more work to set up. If you are unable to design and implement a teaching programme whilst at medical school, do not worry. The golden time to do this is whilst you are a FY1 or FY2. Although your schedule will be jam-packed, there will still be enough time to deliver teaching to medical students who are on placement at your hospital. What is more, these medical students will regularly rotate and a new batch will come in after a certain number of weeks. This means you can recycle the same teaching material for your programme and provide the same learning opportunity for the next cohort of students. To set up teaching, you should contact the undergraduate education team at your Trust and work with them to find the best time and place to deliver your teaching programme.

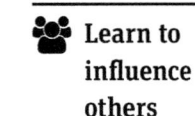

> **Learn to influence others**

Teaching programmes can involve classroom teaching, ward-based teaching, virtual teaching, or even creating electronic learning modules. Again, it is imperative to collect feedback from attendees and gain a signed letter from a senior colleague who is aware of the programme. As before, the signed letter should include information regarding how often you delivered the teaching and what time period this covered. The signed letter should also state that you have identified a gap in the curriculum and have worked with local tutors to design and organise the delivery of your teaching programme.

8.3 Teaching qualifications

In addition to gaining credit for contributing to an existing teaching programme or designing and implementing one, you can also gain credit for completing formal qualifications in teaching. This includes undertaking teaching training courses, a Master's in medical education, or a higher qualification in teaching, such as PGCert or PGDip (many universities and colleges across the UK offer these so look around to see which ones are most appealing). Generally speaking, full-time courses will take a year to complete and the part-time courses tend to take 2 years. You may be interested in pursuing one of these qualifications as part of a teaching fellowship job during a FY3 year (for more information see *Chapter 13*). To gain credit for these qualifications you must evidence an original certificate of attendance. A written reflection on the learning is also advised as supplementary evidence.

If completing a formal qualification like a Master's in medical education or PGCert or PGDip does not appeal to you, it is still possible to gain points in this section by simply attending teaching courses. Bear in mind that some medical schools or foundation schools or Trusts offer dedicated teaching days for free and, if that is the case, keep a record of this in the form of a letter or certificate. Even if your medical school or place of work does not offer you any training in teaching, you do not have to spend too much money – there are some free online courses such as those from the Open University (➤ www.open.edu/openlearn/free-courses/full-catalogue).

To gain more points in this section of your portfolio you must evidence 'substantial training in teaching' which is defined as "**more** than the usual short (1 or 2 day) course which is mandatory for most trainee doctors, and more than the usual online modules completed in a few hours". If you are applying for core surgery, this means you must undergo formal training lasting between 5 and 20 days (whole time equivalent). Recruiters specify that to meet this criterion, you are allowed to attend multiple courses, providing that these courses are complementary and not covering similar topics. Some examples of courses are:

- Teach the teacher courses, e.g. Oxford Medical, Erudical, and ISC Medical.
- The Royal College of Physicians offer various courses, e.g. Effective Teaching Skills, On-the-job teaching, and Work-based assessment.
- The Royal College of Surgeons offer Training the Trainers: Developing Teaching Skills.

Note that these courses cost hundreds of pounds, but it is possible to be reimbursed through your study budget when you are in a training job as a FY2 and above. These courses also fill up very quickly, especially just before IMT and CST applications begin (around November) so look into them early! If you are interested in immersing yourself further into the world of medical education, there are two organisations to be aware of: the Academy of Medical Educators (AoME) and the Association for the Study of Medical Education (ASME). These organisations produce professional standards for medical educators to abide by. They also support medical educators by celebrating their achievements and organising regular events and conferences.

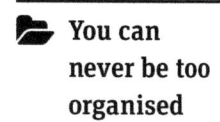

> You can never be too organised

8.4 How points are allocated for teaching others

Tables 8.1–8.4 show how teaching, and training in teaching, points are allocated across internal medical and core surgical training.

Table 8.1: Internal Medicine Training (IMT) 2021 – Teaching experience

Option	Score	Notes
I have worked with local tutors to design and organise a teaching programme (a series of sessions) to enhance locally organised teaching for healthcare professionals or medical students. I have contributed regularly to teaching over a period of approximately 3 months or longer. I have evidence of formal feedback.	6	You have identified a gap in teaching provided and have worked with local tutors to design and organise a teaching programme, and arrange teachers. You have a certificate or letter of recognition for your contribution. You have evidence of formal feedback from these sessions, or a 'Developing the Clinical Teacher' form and have reflected upon this.
I have organised a local teaching programme for healthcare professionals or medical students consisting of more than one session and contributed regularly to teaching over a period of approximately 3 months or longer. I have evidence of formal feedback.	5	You have worked with local tutors to organise an existing programme and arrange teachers. You have a certificate or letter of recognition of your contribution. You have evidence of formal feedback from these sessions, or a 'Developing the Clinical Teacher' form and have reflected upon this.
I have provided regular teaching for healthcare professionals or medical students over a period of approximately 3 months or longer. I have evidence of formal feedback.	3	For example, regular bedside or classroom teaching, acting as a mentor to a student or acting as a tutor in a virtual learning environment. You have a certificate or letter of recognition of your contribution. You have evidence of formal feedback from these sessions, or a 'Developing the Clinical Teacher' form and have reflected upon this.
I have taught medical students or other healthcare professionals occasionally. I have evidence of formal feedback.	2	You have provided teaching on an *ad hoc* basis. You have evidence of formal feedback from these sessions, or a 'Developing the Clinical Teacher' form and have reflected upon this.

Reproduced from ➔ www.imtrecruitment.org.uk/recruitment-process/applying/application-scoring under the Open Government Licence v3.0.

Table 8.2: Core Surgical Training (CST) 2021 – Teaching experience

Option	Score	Notes
I have worked with local tutors to design and organise a teaching programme (a series of sessions) to enhance organised teaching for healthcare professionals or medical students at a regional level AND I have contributed regularly to teaching over a period of approximately 3 months or longer AND I have evidence of formal feedback.	8	You have identified a gap in teaching provided and have worked with local tutors to design and organise a regional teaching programme and arrange teachers.
I have worked with local tutors to design and organise a teaching programme (a series of sessions) to enhance organised teaching for healthcare professionals or medical students at a local level AND I have contributed regularly to teaching over a period of approximately 3 months or longer AND I have evidence of formal feedback.	6	You have identified a gap in teaching provided and have worked with local tutors to design and organise a local teaching programme and arrange teachers.
I have provided regular teaching for healthcare professionals or medical students over a period of approximately 3 months or longer AND I have evidence of formal feedback.	4	For example, regular bedside or classroom teaching, acting as a mentor to a student or acting as a tutor in a virtual learning environment.
I have taught medical students or other healthcare professionals occasionally AND I have evidence of formal feedback.	2	
I have taught medical students or other healthcare professionals occasionally, but I have no formal feedback	1	If you have no formal feedback then you must upload a 200–250 word reflection on your teaching experience to the evidence verification portal.

Reproduced from the *2021 Core Surgical Training Self-Assessment Scoring Guidance for Candidates* handbook (available at ➤ https://coresurgeryinterview.com/resources/2021-Self-Assessment-Guidance-for-Candidates..pdf) under the Open Government Licence v3.0.

TEACHING OTHERS

Table 8.3: Internal Medicine Training (IMT) 2021 – Training in teaching

Option	Score	Notes
I have been awarded a Master's level teaching qualification.	4	This could be full-time over one academic year or part-time over multiple years.
I have a higher qualification in teaching, e.g. PGCert or PGDip.	3	
I have had substantial training in teaching methods lasting more than 2 days; this could include a completed module which forms part of a postgraduate teaching qualification.	2	This should be additional to any training received as part of your primary medical qualification.
I have had brief training in teaching methods lasting no more than 2 days.	1	This should be additional to any training received as part of your primary medical qualification.

Reproduced from ↗ www.imtrecruitment.org.uk/recruitment-process/applying/application-scoring under the Open Government Licence v3.0.

Table 8.4: Core Surgical Training (CST) 2021 – Training in teaching

Option	Score	Notes
I have a Master's level or higher qualification in teaching, e.g. PGCert or PGDip.	4	This could be full-time over one academic year or part-time over multiple years.
I have had substantial training in teaching methods lasting between 5 and 20 days; this could include a completed module which forms part of a postgraduate teaching qualification AND I can provide evidence for this.	3	This should be additional to any training received as part of your primary medical qualification.
I am currently undertaking a course for a higher qualification in teaching AND I can provide evidence to demonstrate this.	3	This should be additional to any training received as part of your primary medical qualification.

(continued)

Table 8.4: *(continued)*

Option	Score	Notes
I have had brief training in teaching methods lasting no more than 2 days AND I can provide evidence to demonstrate this.	2	This should be additional to any training received as part of your primary medical qualification.
I have had brief training in teaching via online modules only AND I can provide evidence to demonstrate this.	1	

Reproduced from the *2021 Core Surgical Training Self-Assessment Scoring Guidance for Candidates* handbook (available at ➤ https://coresurgeryinterview.com/resources/2021-Self-Assessment-Guidance-for-Candidates..pdf) under the Open Government Licence v3.0.

8.5 Top tips for medical students

- **Teaching can be mutually beneficial.** When choosing a topic to teach, either show commitment to your preferred specialty or select a topic that you would benefit from brushing up on.

- **Do not wait around.** As a foundation doctor who is looking to establish a teaching programme for medical students, make sure to get your foot in the door early (medical students have a busy schedule and some of your FY1/FY2 colleagues will want to get in ahead of you).

- **Teaching does not have to be lecture based.** Think outside the box!

- **Teaching can take place anywhere.** It can be done in a doctor's office, the ward, or even your own living room.

- **Make it a multiple part series** and satisfy the timeline requirements to gain points for your portfolio.

- **Collect feedback and act upon it.** It looks good if the feedback gets better over time.

TEACHING OTHERS   CHAPTER 8

- **Inform senior staff members,** i.e. let someone senior to you (e.g. your educational supervisor) know what teaching you are doing so they can provide you with a signed letter once it is all done.
- **Use a template to create your feedback forms.** The Royal College of Physicians and the Royal College of Surgeons provide templates on their websites:
    - www.jrcptb.org.uk/documents/evaluation-form-teaching-and-presentations
    - www.rcseng.ac.uk/education-and-exams/accreditation/participant-feedback-questionnaire/
- Consider using the feedback that you collect to design a study.

> Always have a plan

8.6 Advice from the experts

Professor Chloe Orkin:

"Try to put yourself in the position of the audience. What would you like to learn if you were sitting in the front row? Make fantastic slides, make it visual. Use humour. Try to find your own voice and be yourself. Know your slides – don't be as surprised as the audience when seeing your next slide!!"

Dr Elaine Winkley:

"Start early, get involved, and work with non-doctor groups, i.e. allied healthcare professionals. Look beyond the obvious."

Mr Gareth Dobson:

"Be proactive. Opportunities to teach are endless, whether this is informal ward teaching, organised regional sessions or national teaching sessions. People generally do not turn down offers of teaching and, with a little organisation and preparation, you can easily set up teaching sessions. My top tip would be, don't forget nursing and allied healthcare colleagues – in my experience they're incredibly keen and grateful for teaching sessions and, equally, can teach you valuable things in return."

Dr George Miller:

"Gaining the opportunity to teach is very straightforward once you've taken on roles within university societies; just endeavour to always collect feedback."

Dr Jeeves Wijesuriya:

"As an academic whose background is largely in medical education, I would say that it's worth thinking about getting some formal training in medical education and its fundamentals. Practically, teaching in clinical contexts is about identifying where there is a need and how you can help. Given we all work in a peer-led apprenticeship-style system, there are loads of opportunities to teach colleagues. Whether that's teaching undergraduate students theory, or practising OSCEs or working with other more junior colleagues, we can really contribute to teaching. The key is using these opportunities to both develop our own teaching practice and recording it. Something as simple as feedback sheets or questionnaires can help, so do both. Through collecting feedback, you deliver for a portfolio and give yourself an opportunity to learn and improve your teaching content and style. There are, of course, also formal courses and clinical teaching that takes place on the ward, and never enough clinicians to help take part. This is again where being keen to volunteer can help! Medical schools are often looking for examiners, invigilators or people to help with OSCE teaching. Emailing your local medical school as a foundation doctor or even your medical education department in the hospital can identify some great opportunities."

> **HOMEWORK 9:**
>
> Keep your eyes open to see if you can identify a gap in the medical school curriculum. Think about how you can effectively deliver teaching to fill this gap. Consider the timeline that will be involved and how you will regularly achieve an audience. Reach out to faculty for help and let someone (e.g. your supervisor) know what you are doing.

✏️ Always have a plan

CHAPTER 9

Quality improvement

Quality improvement in healthcare refers to the process of making positive changes in the workplace and this can include almost anything. Some of the common domains for improvement are patient/staff safety, patient/staff satisfaction, cost-effectiveness, efficiency, and equitability. For the improvement to be classed as a quality improvement (QI) project, it must abide by QI methodology, i.e. the **Plan, Do, Study Act (PDSA) cycle**:

1. **Plan** – this involves identifying an area for improvement and deciding the best way to measure the current performance. It also involves forming a team if necessary.
2. **Do** – this involves data collection of parameters such as current performance, opinions of potential change, and associated costs.
3. **Study** – this involves data analysis, i.e. recognising trends in data, comparing these trends to what you predicted, and beginning to develop a strategy for improvement.
4. **Act** – this involves implementing the improvement.

Completion of all four steps is referred to as completing one PDSA cycle. The process should then be repeated (i.e. a second PDSA cycle should be completed) to confirm if your improvement has actually achieved its desired effect (you should set a target outcome). If it has not, and the impact of your improvement falls short of your target, you should complete another PDSA cycle. The process of carrying out further PDSA cycles should continue until the set target has been met.

QI projects are tremendously valuable to organisations across all sectors. Hence it is so important to have an impressive QI project under your belt, regardless of what career path you favour. In healthcare, QI projects are very heavily weighted when applicants are considered for a specialty position. In fact, there are usually more points up for grabs in this category of your portfolio than in any other. Participating in a QI project has even become a mandatory component of passing FY1 and FY2. For medical students, it is never too early for you to become involved in a QI project. If you are allocated to a consultant on a particular ward, express your interest in becoming involved in a QI project and attempt to identify potential areas for improvement on the ward. It may be something as simple as putting up a whiteboard in every bay and writing the date, weather outside, and a news headline for patients to read. Completing multiple PDSA cycles involving simple patient satisfaction surveys might show improvement. There may also be some interesting hypotheses to investigate related to patients' cognition. This is an example you may wish to adapt. However, bear in mind that the best QI projects are ones that solve a significant problem that you have encountered.

If you do not become involved in a QI project whilst at medical school, do not worry. When you start work and become very familiar with a department, you will begin to notice areas for improvement. We guarantee it! If you would like some further information on quality improvement, here are some very useful websites for you to visit:

- www.health.org.uk/sites/default/files/QualityImprovementMadeSimple.pdf
- www.bmj.com/content/364/bmj.k5437
- www.kingsfund.org.uk/publications/making-case-quality-improvement
- www.hqip.org.uk
- www.ihi.org.

If quality improvement is something that you are particularly interested in, there are opportunities to gain formal training and qualifications. For example, Health Education England South West has announced a training opportunity for doctors to work with senior staff on QI and to gain a postgraduate qualification (PGCert) in Health Services Improvement with Exeter University.

Now that we understand the process of completing a QI project, it is important to appreciate the level of participation you must evidence to maximise the strength of your portfolio. Recruiters need to see that you have played a lead role in designing the QI project, implementing the QI methodology (PDSA cycles), and identifying sustainability for the work. This is typically evidenced by a signed letter from your supervisor. It is noteworthy that for specialty job applications you will not be able to claim points in the presentations section of the application for presenting a QI project (unless you present more than one).

> You can never be too organised

QUALITY IMPROVEMENT   CHAPTER 9

9.1 How points are allocated for quality improvement

Tables 9.1 and *9.2* show the points awarded across internal medical and core surgical training.

Table 9.1: Internal Medicine Training (IMT) 2021 – Quality improvement

Option	Score	Notes
Involvement in all stages of three or more cycles of a QI project	8	For example, you participated in all stages of two PDSA cycles (or similar) as well as a further cycle consisting, as a minimum, of data collection and analysis.
		Involvement in a project where a change/act/action step has not been carried out but only suggestions for change created/presented does not constitute involvement in all stages.
		Presentation of a project is not an essential stage as not all QI work requires presentation.
		It is likely that this involved working as part of a team, but you must evidence your own role within the QI activity for all stages.
Involvement in all stages of two cycles of a QI project	6	For example, you participated in all stages of a PDSA cycle (or similar) as well as a further cycle consisting, as a minimum, of data collection and analysis.
Involvement in some stages of two or more cycles of a QI project	4	For example, you were involved in data collection/analysis for two cycles of a QI project but not the change and/or planning stages.
Involved in all stages of a single cycle of a QI project	4	For example, you participated in all stages of a PDSA cycle or were involved in planning, data collection, data analysis, and change.
Involvement in some stages of a single cycle of a QI project	2	For example, you were involved in data collection and analysis or a project that didn't implement any change.

Reproduced from ➔ www.imtrecruitment.org.uk/recruitment-process/applying/application-scoring under the Open Government Licence v3.0.

Table 9.2: Core Surgical Training (CST) 2021 – Quality improvement

Option	Score	Notes
I played a leading role in the design and implementation of a sustainable change (i.e. more than one completed cycle) using QI methodology or clinical audit AND I have presented the complete results at a regional or national meeting	11	You had a lead role in devising the question to be asked (or how an existing project could be developed further/sustained), developing the project plan, identifying potential solutions, implementing repeated change cycles, collating and presenting the data and identifying sustainability for the work. It is likely that this involved working as part of a team, but you must evidence your own role within the QI activity with demonstrable leadership in design, implementation and learning.
I played a leading role in the design and implementation of a sustainable change (i.e. more than one completed cycle) using QI methodology or clinical audit AND I have presented the complete results at a local meeting	9	As above, but presented within a locality/organisation (e.g. NHS Trust, hospital, primary care network).
I played a leading role in the design and implementation of a sustainable change (i.e. more than one completed cycle) using QI methodology or clinical audit, but I have not presented the results	8	As above; but the work was not presented by you.
I have actively participated in the design and implementation of a sustainable change (i.e. more than one completed cycle) using QI methodology or clinical audit, AND I have presented the complete results at a meeting	6	You participated actively through multiple cycles and presented the findings, but did not take a leading role in the project.
I have actively participated in the design and implementation of a sustainable (i.e. more than one completed cycle) change using QI methodology or clinical audit, but I have not presented the complete results at a meeting	4	You participated actively in the project through multiple cycles but did not take a leading role or present the findings.
I have participated only in certain stages of a QI project or clinical audit, which has completed at least one cycle	2	For example, you assisted with data collection for the project.

Reproduced from the *2021 Core Surgical Training Self-Assessment Scoring Guidance for Candidates* handbook (available at ↗ https://coresurgeryinterview.com/resources/2021-Self-Assessment-Guidance-for-Candidates..pdf) under the Open Government Licence v3.0.

9.2 Top tips for medical students

- **You can only claim points for one QI project in the QI section of your portfolio**, so once you have chosen to start one, give it your all.
- **Visit the website of NHS Trusts** and see if they provide case studies of successful QI projects e.g. https://bethechangeasph.com. These can be used for inspiration.
- **Try to choose something that interests you.**
- **Do not be afraid to involve those around you and ask for advice.**
- **Data collection can be an arduous process.** Try to make it as easy for yourself as possible. Strategies for this include building a team of reliable people, only measuring valuable parameters, and utilising online survey tools, e.g. Google Forms.
- **Create a draft letter** that describes your involvement in the QI project and ask your supervisor to sign it. Make sure this letter includes accurate wording, so you are able to claim all of the points you are entitled to.

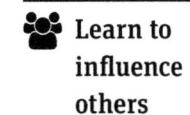

Learn to influence others

9.3 Advice from the experts

Professor Chloe Orkin:

"Keep your eyes peeled. If something needs improving, suggest a QI project and offer to lead or help."

Dr Elaine Winkley:

"Get involved in projects you can commit time and enthusiasm to and choose mentors wisely. You want to be with people that can drive change and get things finished and moved forward."

Mr Gareth Dobson:

"Keep it realistic. It's often difficult to appreciate the working of a department during a short placement. I utilised supervisors to discuss potential ideas for quality improvement projects. One key thing I would suggest is to make sure the project is achievable in the time frame you have allocated."

Dr George Miller:

"There are lots of opportunities on the ward. If possible close the loop on previous audits that have been conducted by doctors or medical students on the ward before you. It will save you time, be of greater utility, and gain you points on your applications."

Dr Jeeves Wijesuriya:

"Quality improvement projects are largely based on a simple premise: identifying something that you think could be done better. As a medical student or junior doctor you will identify loads of these situations in your day-to-day life on the wards or in practices. Whether it's something as simple as adding bookmarks to medical notes to speed up ward rounds, or changing the way discharges work across a Trust, all quality improvement starts with identifying an issue, quantifying it with data and then finding an intervention and seeing if it improves these outcomes. Most senior clinicians will welcome someone with an idea or even if simply keen and happy to help with a project they may have. The key is to ask."

> **HOMEWORK 10:**
>
> Express your interest in developing a QI project to your supervisor. When in a clinical setting, begin to consider potential improvements that could be made and measured.

Always have a plan

CHAPTER 10

Demonstrating commitment

Demonstrating commitment is the sixth and final piece of the portfolio jigsaw. It may be unclear to you which career path you want to pursue, but there are simple ways you can demonstrate commitment to a broad spectrum of careers. If you already know the career path for you, there are some additional methods for you to consider.

10.1 Ways to demonstrate commitment

In this chapter we cover the eight most common ways for medical students and foundation doctors to show commitment to a career path. This is not an exhaustive list and almost all of the topics we have already discussed can be re-applied to this category. Our aim is to signpost some of the extra components that medical students and junior doctors may not otherwise have thought of.

10.1.1 Logbooks

A logbook is a written record of your activity that is displayed in a table. Our advice to medical students is to create a digital logbook as soon as possible and to update it every time you attend a surgical procedure or specialist clinic. The rationale for keeping a logbook is that it allows you to evidence your experience and interest in a specialty. Even if you do not know what specialty you would like to pursue, there is a strong likelihood that a comprehensive logbook of all your attendances in theatres/clinics will be of significant value to you in the future. Logbooks are easy to update and do not require a lot of detail (see our example of a logbook entry in *Table 10.1*). It is essential to have your logbook signed off by each supervisor so that they can validate your activity. Our advice is to print off your logbook at the end of a rotation and ask your supervisor to sign and date it. Some written feedback from your supervisor would also be a useful addition. There are many logbook websites that allow you to do all of this online (e.g. www.elogbook.org).

> You can never be too organised

Table 10.1: Example logbook entry

Session number, date, time	Procedure/ presenting complaint	Case notes	Observations and learning	Location	Supervisor
Session 1, 20/11/2020, Afternoon	Corneal cross-link procedure	26-year-old male patient with keratoconus	I observed the procedure and gained an understanding of corneal cross-linking	Eye theatre, Whiston Hospital	Miss Butt *Butt*
Session 2, 15/03/2021, Morning	Nystagmus	9-month-old boy with nystagmus, reduced eye contact and pale complexion	Slit lamp examination: red reflex visible through iris. Diagnosis: Ocular cutaneous albinism. Referral made to dermatology and geneticist for counselling.	Paediatrics outpatients department, Whiston Hospital	Miss Butt *Butt*

10.1.2 Elective

Towards the end of medical school, you will need to complete an elective placement. This is typically a 5–8 week hospital placement which can be anywhere in the world. It is a great way to travel with your close friends and experience healthcare systems in other countries. Depending on your desired elective, you may need to plan quite a long way ahead; for example, South African trauma centres are known to be fully booked years in advance. There are also many adventure-style electives that require extensive planning, such as the Royal Flying Doctor Service of Australia, Himalayan Health Exchange, and jungle medicine on the Amazon Hope.

Electives can be very expensive, and it is a good idea to find out if there are any bursaries or grants you can apply for (see *Section 6.3* for examples). Because you are very close to entering employment, it may also be worthwhile applying for an interest-free credit card.

The process of applying for a medical elective normally involves visiting the website of the organisation you wish to volunteer for and finding an email address to make an enquiry. You must then coordinate everything so that you meet the requirements set by the organisation and your university. Note that there are agencies who can help you with this process, for example:

- **www.electives.net/splash** – free for MDU student members
- **www.projects-abroad.co.uk/medical-electives**
- **http://electives.us** – for electives in the USA
- **www.electiveafrica.com** – for electives in Africa.

Electives are a great opportunity to travel and explore exciting areas of the world. Ensure that you have fun and make lasting memories, but do not forget that electives also enable you to show commitment to a career path in many ways:

- You can keep a logbook of procedures, clinics, and interesting cases.
- You can ask for a signed feedback letter from your supervisor.
- You can become involved in a research or quality improvement project.
- You can write a reflection and present or publish this somewhere.

> *Avoid burnout*

10.1.3 Taster weeks

During FY1 and FY2, junior doctors are granted a combined total of 45 days of study leave (15 days during FY1 and 30 days during FY2). The majority of this will be taken up by mandatory teaching sessions that are provided by your hospital. Depending on how much teaching your hospital provides, the remaining study leave days can be used for learning outside your Trust, e.g. training days (see *Sections 10.1.4*), conferences and exams (see *Section 5.2*). One way that all junior doctors are supposed to use their study leave during FY1 and FY2 is a taster week. This is essentially a week of work experience, which can be done in any hospital and any department. You may even want to do this abroad. To arrange a taster week, you should email a consultant or the head of department where you want to visit. You must then coordinate everything so that you are able to complete your taster week at a time your rota coordinator is happy with. Similar to completing an elective placement, taster weeks allow you to show commitment to a career path in many ways.

> *Always have a plan*

10.1.4 Training courses

Another way that FY1 and FY2 doctors are able to use their remaining study leave is by completing training courses. Depending on what specialty you want to pursue, there should be a list of approved courses on the Royal College website or in portfolio guidance documents. Other courses may still be worthwhile, but approved courses are the ones that gain you points for your future job applications. The types of training courses vary and include surgical skills, clinical skills, education programmes, and anatomy/dissection courses. Training courses can be very expensive, especially if you attend several of them, which is why most junior doctors wait until their FY2 before completing courses. In FY2, junior doctors are able to gain access to study budget money, which can contribute towards these costs. Also, at this stage of their career, junior doctors are more likely to be certain of their desired career path and will be less likely to waste money on a course that does not benefit them. The courses that are available to medical students are much cheaper and if you are strongly inclined to pursue a particular specialty, you should investigate the relevant training courses that are available to you before you graduate. Here are some useful links to help you find courses that are available for medical students and foundation doctors:

- **www.rcplondon.ac.uk/education-practice/courses**
- **www.rcseng.ac.uk/education-and-exams/courses**
- **www.rcgp.org.uk/learning/courses-and-events.aspx**.

10.1.5 Examinations

Another example of utilising study leave is revising for and sitting examinations (see *Section 5.2* for further guidance).

10.1.6 Societies

When applying for a specialty training position, credit is sometimes given to those who have been members of a society (whether as students or junior doctors) that is relevant to that specialty. Examples of medical societies include the Royal Society of Medicine, British Cardiovascular Society, British Maternal and Foetal Medicine Society, and the Royal Society for Public Health. Examples of surgical societies include the Association of Surgeons of Great Britain and Ireland, British Association of Paediatric Surgeons, and Society of British Neurological Surgeons. The membership fees can be expensive but there is often a reduction for students. There may also be competitions open to non-members whereby free membership is awarded to the winner. Once you are a member of a society, you should try to make the most of the access it grants you. In other words, take part in as many training days, teaching sessions, conferences, and competitions as you possibly can. This will give you a great chance of boosting your CV and will give you much to talk about at interview.

10.1.7 Student-selected research projects and rotations

As part of your medical school curriculum, you will complete student-selected research projects and rotations. If you are interested in an area of healthcare or a particular specialty, you should use these student-selected components of the curriculum to explore this interest. As discussed in previous chapters, time spent completing a project or a rotation is a great opportunity for publications, presentations, prizes and awards, and QI projects. However, if you find that by the end of the project or rotation you are unable to pursue any of these, do not worry, because you can still gain credit for demonstrating commitment to that area of healthcare or particular specialty by asking your supervisor for a signed letter. Ideally, this letter will include as much relevant information as possible, such as the title of your project and your overall grade, the length of your rotation and activities you were involved in, and general feedback with gratitude for your contributions. If somehow you take part in a student-selected project or rotation in an area of healthcare or in a specialty that you have no interest in pursuing as a career, our advice is to still request this signed letter. There is a strong likelihood it will be of use to you at some stage in the future.

> ✏️ Always have a plan

10.1.8 Conferences

The best reason to be at a conference is if you are a part of the organising team or if you are presenting work there. Nevertheless, if you find that all of the conferences you have taken part in are associated with specialties you do not want to pursue a career in, or if you have not been able to take part in any conferences thus far, you can still gain credit for attending as a delegate. This shows recruiters that you have an interest in a particular area of healthcare and are willing to take time out of your schedule to learn and network. To ensure that you gain credit for this, you should keep evidence of your attendance, e.g. certificate or ID badge. We also advise you to attach a written reflection on what you were able to gain from your attendance. See *Section 5.3.6* for information on presenting work at conferences and also for a list of websites that can help you to find future conferences.

10.2 How points are allocated for demonstrating commitment

There are no points available for demonstrating commitment to specialty in Internal Medicine Training (IMT) 2021, but *Table 10.2* shows those available in core surgical training.

Table 10.2: Core Surgical Training (CST) 2021 – Commitment to specialty

Option	Score	Notes
MRCS Part A Examination: choose one of the following options		
I have sat and passed the MRCS Part A Examination	3	Examples include: email or PDF showing a pass in MRCS Part A
I have sat and failed the MRCS Part A Examination OR I have already booked to sit the exam in the future	1	Examples include: email confirmation showing exam booked for January 2021 or email showing failed exam
Attendance at surgical courses: choose one of the following options		
I have attended 2 or more surgical courses	4	Proof of attendance must be provided
I have attended 1 surgical course	2	Proof of attendance must be provided
Surgical experience: choose one of the following options		
Involvement in 15 cases or more	3	
Involvement in 11-14 cases	2	
Involvement in 5-10 cases	1	
Completion of a surgical taster: choose one of the following options		
I have attended 4–5 days of surgical taster sessions	3	Reflection required
I have attended 1–3 days of surgical taster sessions	1	Reflection required
Completion of a surgical elective: choose one of the following options		
I have undertaken an elective in a surgical specialty	3	Reflection required

Reproduced from the *2021 Core Surgical Training Self-Assessment Scoring Guidance for Candidates* handbook (available at **https://coresurgeryinterview.com/resources/2021-Self-Assessment-Guidance-for-Candidates..pdf**) under the Open Government Licence v3.0.

Despite the fact that no points are available for IMT applicants, demonstrating commitment towards medicine may play a significant role in IMT interviews. It will also play a large role for IMT doctors when applying for Specialist Training (ST) further down the line. Note that demonstrating commitment plays a major role in applications to run-through programmes (see *Section 14.4*).

10.3 Top tips for medical students

- **Create a logbook as soon as you can and keep it updated.** If you attend multiple procedures or clinics in one day, it can be difficult to remember all of the details for your logbook and so make notes on your phone after each procedure or clinic.

- **Consider what type of elective you want to go on.** Plan well in advance and attempt to become involved in a project that can be used for publication or competitions.

- **Arrange taster weeks early.** The earlier you are able to perform a taster week, the longer you have to work alongside that department to complete projects and to publish or present them.

- **Visit Royal College websites** of specialties that you are interested in to see if there are any courses available for you to attend.

- **Use student-selected projects and rotations wisely.** They can gain you a lot of credit if you are able to achieve a publication or presentation. Always request a signed letter from your supervisor (that you have drafted).

- **Keep evidence of your attendance at conferences.**

10.4 Advice from the experts

Professor Chloe Orkin:

"Try to go beyond just doing your day job."

Dr Elaine Winkley:

"Grasp opportunities, ask for taster days, contact people, ask around colleagues and tutors and get them to link you up with those in the relevant specialty. Be prepared to use your own time to get the exposure you need."

Mr Gareth Dobson:

"Don't panic if you're not sure. If you have an idea early on what specialty you are interested in then great, introduce yourself to some of the team and see if you can get involved with a project. If you don't know, don't panic. As long as you have a balanced CV and a genuine reason for pursuing a career in that specialty then you should be okay."

Dr George Miller:

"By involving yourself in university societies, publishing and teaching, you will have ample opportunity to demonstrate your commitment to your specialty."

Dr Jeeves Wijesuriya:

"The first step is to look at getting experience in that specialty, whether that's through selected modules, joining specialty societies at medical school, taster weeks, or jobs in foundation training – the key is showing you have worked in and understand the specialty. If you look at trainee societies or Royal College websites, they will often have committees, fellowships, scholarships or free places at courses or conferences that will also enable you to get more understanding of the specialty and be able to demonstrate experience! I highly recommend the simple step of Googling and exploring Royal College and trainee group websites as they will be full of information and advice about applications and experience! One of the best examples is the Association of Surgeons in Training website (**www.asit.org/resources/medical-students**) which has loads on experience, applications and bursaries to help prospective surgeons with their applications."

> You can never be too organised

> **HOMEWORK 11:**
>
> Make a logbook and keep it updated. If you are yet to go on your elective, investigate the many different options and plan ahead. Doctors love talking about their electives, so do not be afraid to ask them for information and contact details.

CHAPTER 11

General tips for building your portfolio

Now that we have covered all six aspects of your portfolio, here are the key things for you to remember when attempting to build it effectively.

- **Become familiarised with the points system for portfolio self-assessment.**
- **Try to kill multiple birds with one stone**, for example, intercalating in a Master's, getting your dissertation published, presenting the findings at a conference, evidencing your efforts to win a prize or award. This excludes QI projects, for which you are only allowed to gain points in one category.
- **Collaborate wisely.** Find consultants and registrars who are interested in research and have a proven track record for helping students gain publications and presentations. Stay in contact with them and enquire about further projects.
- **Cast the net out for opportunities.** Take some time to write formal emails that can be sent to doctors. These emails should declare your admiration for their work, and they should express your interest in following in their footsteps. Explain that you wish to become involved in projects that will boost your portfolio. Don't forget to mention the qualities that you will bring to the table.
- **Always try to take your projects one step further** and gain points for future job applications. If you completed a project a while ago and did not make the most of it, revisit the project and see if it can be recycled into something that will gain you points.
- Remember, to a very large extent, the area of healthcare or specialty associated with your project **does not matter**.

You will not miss out on any points for your job applications if your projects are about other specialties. Recruiters want to see that you are capable of getting projects over the finishing line. If it is related to the specialty you are applying for, that is merely a bonus.

- **Use LinkedIn for inspiration**. Find doctors that have impressive profiles and see what steps they have taken to reach their current position. LinkedIn will tell you about their research, prizes and awards, exams, fellowships, voluntary positions, etc.

- **Request confirmation letters**. It is very important to receive signed letters for activities that will add to your portfolio. These should be signed by your supervisor and include an appropriate amount of detail. Never be afraid to draft your own letter and to ask your supervisor to sign it. That way you can include the specific wording that is required to gain all of the points you are entitled to. As long as what you have written is accurate, your supervisor will be appreciative.

- **Create a pdf copy of all of your evidence documents and store them safely.**

CHAPTER 12

The foundation programme (FY1 and FY2)

There are four foundation programmes that final year medical students can apply to:
- Standard UK Foundation Programme
- Academic Foundation Programme (AFP)
- Foundation Priority Programme (FPP)
- Psychiatry Foundation Fellowship (PFF) Programme.

12.1 Standard UK foundation programme

You must apply for the standard UK Foundation Programme even if you also intend to apply for the AFP and/or FPP and/or PFF. Early on in your final year at medical school you will receive emails from your medical school faculty about setting up an Oriel account. Oriel is the website (➤ www.oriel.nhs.uk) that the NHS uses to allocate jobs to doctors. The standard UK Foundation Programme uses a points-based system for applications, whereby **the maximum number of Foundation Programme Application System (FPAS) points for an applicant is 100.**

The score comprises two elements:
1. Educational Performance Measure (EPM): **maximum 50 points**
2. Situational Judgement Test: **maximum 50 points**

12.1.1 Educational performance measure

The EPM points that are up for grabs can be broken down as follows:

Medical school performance:
- maximum = 43 FPAS points
- minimum = 34 FPAS points

This is based on what decile you fall into, i.e. what 10% band of the year group your overall exam/assessment performance at medical school equates to (e.g. you may fall into the top 10% of the year, or the top 20% of the year, etc.). Your medical school provides this information to the Oriel system. If you are in the first decile (i.e. the top 10% of your year) you will receive a score of 43. If you are in the second decile, your score will be 42, and so on. This continues until those who are in the tenth decile (i.e. the bottom 10% of the year) receive the minimum score of 34.

Additional degrees:
- maximum = 5 FPAS points
- minimum = 0 FPAS points

For the most part this includes intercalation degrees and, if you are a postgraduate student, degrees before starting medicine. It is your responsibility to provide this information on your Oriel application, along with appropriate evidence (see below). You can receive up to **5 points** for your additional degree (see *Table 12.1*), but you will score 0 points if you have no additional degrees. You can only claim for one degree even if you have more than one. Therefore, you must ensure that you claim for the additional degree that will give you the highest number of points.

Table 12.1: FPAS points available for additional degrees

FPAS points	Qualification
0	• Primary medical qualification only • 3rd class BMedSci integrated course
1	• 3rd class honours degree • Unclassified honours degree • 2.2 class BMedSci integrated course
2	• 2.2 class honours degree • 2.1 class BMedSci integrated course
3	• 2.1 class honours degree • 1st class BMedSci integrated course
4	• 1st class honours degree • Postgraduate Master's degree (level 7 only), e.g. MPhil, MSc, MPharm • Bachelor of Dental Surgery (BDS) • Bachelor of Veterinary Medicine (B Vet Med)
5	• Doctoral degree (e.g. PhD, DPhil, etc.)

Adapted from UK Foundation Programme UKFP 2021 Applicants' Handbook.

Applicants must upload a scanned copy of their original certificate onto Oriel in order to gain these points. If you have not received your original certificate yet (as is often the case with those who have intercalated in a Master's degree), you must upload a letter of confirmation that has been written on university headed paper and is signed by the Dean or a senior authority in the Registrar's office. Make sure you request this well in advance of the deadline, which is usually sometime in October. There have been many cases in which this letter has not been provided before the deadline and so the candidates were unable to claim these FPAS points.

> You can never be too organised

Publications:
- maximum = 2 FPAS points
- minimum = 0 FPAS points

These need to be already published pieces of work that have PubMed ID numbers and you need to be a listed author on the paper (you receive no points as a collaborator). It is your responsibility to provide this information on Oriel with evidence. You can claim a maximum of two points for two publications (one point awarded for each).

> **Note:** *We highly recommend that you thoroughly read the most up-to-date UK Foundation Programme Applicants' Handbook to ensure that you receive all the points you deserve.*

12.1.2 Situational judgement test

The SJT is an exam that lasts for 2 hours and 20 minutes. The exam takes place during your final year of medical school and you will have only one opportunity to sit it, in either December or January; some medical schools choose when you sit the exam, others give you the option to sit it on the date you prefer. Each SJT question provides a clinical scenario and a list of multiple-choice answers. The question will ask you to either:

1. Rank in order the five answers, e.g. 1 = most appropriate; 5 = least appropriate
2. Select the three answers that are most correct when combined.

The theme of the exam is to test your ability as a prospective foundation doctor to ensure optimal patient safety (without testing your clinical knowledge). A panel of junior doctors and consultants determine the answers to the questions. You will notice throughout your preparations that the answers are somewhat subjective. It is therefore very difficult to revise for this exam and improve your score.

However, there are some ways to prepare yourself to the best of your abilities.

- For general guidance, visit these online resources:
  - **www.foundationprogramme.nhs.uk/faqs/situational-judgement-test-sjt-faqs**
  - **www.geekymedics.com/top-tips-for-the-situational-judgement-test-sjt**

- For practice questions there are two official past papers that can be accessed online at **www.foundationprogramme.nhs.uk/situational-judgement-test-sjt/practice-sjt-papers**. A free online question bank is available at **https://medibuddy.co.uk/foundation/sjt-question-bank/list/**. There are also some inexpensive online question banks that you might find helpful, e.g. **www.pastest.com** and **www.onexamination.com**. Some question bank websites provide combination subscription packages, which can be used to also prepare for medical school finals and the Prescribing Safety Assessment (PSA), e.g. **www.passmedicine.com**, and so they may offer better value for money.

- There are SJT crash courses that you can attend, e.g. MDU £75, Emedica £99, and Medset £89. These courses usually sell out around September–October. The general feedback from doctors who have attended these courses is positive; they offer a useful introduction to the SJT and help with aspects such as nervousness and time management. However, feedback from doctors also suggests that they are unlikely to significantly improve your score.

We advise not to over-prepare for the SJT. Sometimes the best way to answer a question is to go with your gut rather than overthink it. Having said this, you ought to know the structure and have had at least one go at the official practice papers! Time is of the essence in this exam so try to pace yourself when attempting practice papers. You should not hang too much hope on the SJT and instead you should focus on claiming as many Oriel points for medical school performance, additional degrees, and publications as you possibly can. The spread of SJT scores across the UK corresponds to a bell-shaped curve. The vast majority of scores will be close to the average (usually around 40) and only a minority will deviate significantly. After you have received your score for the SJT, this is combined with your EPM score to provide a total score out of 100 FPAS points.

Avoid burnout

THE FOUNDATION PROGRAMME (FY1 AND FY2)   CHAPTER 12

12.1.3 Foundation school selection

Each foundation school has an agreed number of positions for applicants and the higher your overall score, the more likely you are to get your top choice location and rotations. Some foundation schools are more competitive to enter than others (particularly the London ones). The 20 foundation schools are as shown in *Figure 12.1*.

Note: *Over the years, some of these foundation schools have changed/merged so check before you rank your choices!*

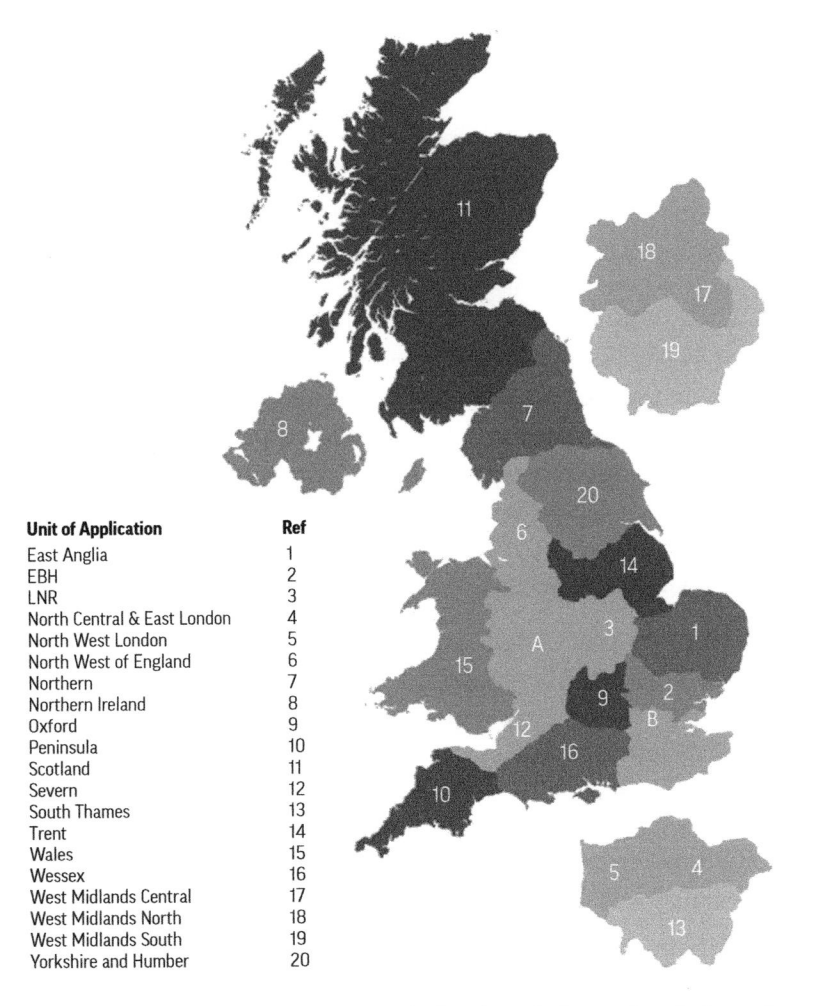

Figure 12.1: Geographical distribution of foundation schools.

Reproduced from UK Foundation Programme UKFP 2021 Applicant's Handbook with permission.

Unit of Application	Ref
East Anglia	1
EBH	2
LNR	3
North Central & East London	4
North West London	5
North West of England	6
Northern	7
Northern Ireland	8
Oxford	9
Peninsula	10
Scotland	11
Severn	12
South Thames	13
Trent	14
Wales	15
Wessex	16
West Midlands Central	17
West Midlands North	18
West Midlands South	19
Yorkshire and Humber	20

The deadline for candidates to rank the foundation schools in order of preference is usually during the first week of November. Typically during the first week of March (after all EPM scores have been added to SJT scores to provide total FPAS points), Oriel will allocate each candidate to a foundation school. This process begins from the

87

candidate with the highest total points and ends with the candidate who has scored the lowest. Oriel will attempt to give everyone their first choice, but if that foundation school is already full, they will move down your list of preferences until there is a vacancy. In a situation where there are more applicants than foundation posts, those below the cut-off will be placed on the reserve list. There may be candidates who are unable to take up their foundation post due to personal circumstances and their places will therefore be offered to someone on the reserve list. If you are unsuccessful in gaining a post, do not lose faith. Instead, work to strengthen your application for next year!

Special circumstances

It may possible to be pre-allocated to your preferred foundation school (regardless of your points) based on your special circumstances, e.g. if you are the primary carer for a close relative, or if you require ongoing medical follow-up that is only available in a specific region, or you have other educational or unique circumstances. If you believe that you qualify for special circumstances, speak with your medical school faculty to receive support throughout the application process. To receive pre-allocation based on special circumstances, you will have to complete a separate electronic form from the UKFPO website:

➤ **www.foundationprogramme.nhs.uk/resources/ 2-year-foundation-programme-documents**.

Linking applications

If you and another person would like to be allocated to the same foundation school, it is possible for your applications to be linked. To do this, you must supply each other's email addresses to Oriel and rank all of your preferences in the same order. You will then be allocated to a foundation school based on the points of the person who has the lowest total. Once allocated to a foundation school, there is no guarantee that you will later be allocated to the same region within that foundation school or the same NHS Trust.

12.1.4 Tracks

After you have been allocated to a foundation school, you must then rank all of the 'tracks' within it. A track is a summary of a candidate's FY1 rotations and FY2 rotations (see *Table 12.2*).

Table 12.2: Example track

FY1 – St George's Hospital			FY2 – St George's Hospital		
Colorectal surgery	Rheumatology	Geriatrics	Renal medicine	A&E	GP

Each foundation school has a unique number of tracks for you to rank. However, it is likely that you will need to rank hundreds of tracks within a short time frame. It is difficult to rank all the available options well and accurately without a strategy. Our advice is to download an Excel copy of the list of tracks and to create an extra column entitled 'overall score'. You should then apply your own scoring system to the tracks and use Excel to arrange the tracks according to their overall score. This is the most systematic and time efficient way of arranging the tracks. *Table 12.3* shows a simple example of a scoring system that you may wish to adopt.

> Always have a plan

Table 12.3: Potential point scoring system

Score awarded for each hospital				
Very preferable hospital = +2	Preferable hospital = +1	Indifferent hospital = 0	Undesirable hospital = –1	Very undesirable hospital = –2
Score awarded for each rotation				
Very preferable rotation = +2	Preferable rotation = +1	Indifferent rotation = 0	Undesirable rotation = –1	Very undesirable rotation = –2

Similarly to the process of allocating candidates to foundation schools, Oriel will begin with the candidate who has the highest overall points and attempt to give everyone their first choice. If a candidate's first choice has already been taken, Oriel will move down that candidate's list of preferences until there is a vacancy.

12.1.5 Some things to consider when ranking destinations

- **Simply rank in terms of preference.** There is no benefit in trying to be tactical. A list of minimum entry scores from previous years can be found on the foundation programme website. Some candidates would prefer to be one of the highest points scorers in their foundation school rather than one of the lowest scorers and so they may adjust their list of foundation school preferences. Our advice is to avoid this, because every year the minimum entry score will vary. Also, even if you are one of the lowest scorers in the foundation school, you may still be given a preferable track, as everyone ranks the tracks differently.

- **Do not be afraid to spread your wings.** You are only signing up for a 2-year commitment and have a licence to roam anywhere in the UK. FY1 and FY2 is a great excuse to discover a new city and make new friends.

- **Account for the cost of living.** If you have spent some time away from home during medical school, you might enjoy moving back if this is an option. Some cities in the UK are very expensive to live in. 'London banding' pay is given to those that work in and around the capital, but this is not enough to cover the extra costs.

- **Consider access to opportunities.** Although London is very expensive, it is the hub for many of the country's leading research centres, Royal Colleges and Societies, conferences, training courses, and so on. Having said this, there are various tertiary centres of excellence depending on the specialty across the UK, so don't just focus on London merely for this reason!

- **Discover the intricacies of every foundation school.** For example, South Thames is split into four sub-sections: link 1, link 2, link 3 and continuity. For links 1, 2, and 3 each track consists of a 'year in' London and a 'year out' of London (though note that your 'year in' can still be far away from London city centre and your 'year out' can still be very much in the heart of it!). Each link contains hospitals according to their geography, i.e. link 1 is westerly, link 2 is central, and link 3 is easterly. Continuity allows candidates to stay in close proximity for their FY1 and FY2. South Thames foundation school, as well as some of the other foundation schools, runs a 'swap shop' during FY1, which gives doctors the chance to swap their FY2 rotations (if in the same Trust) or their entire FY2 year.

- The whole of Wales, Scotland and Northern Ireland are each foundation schools (yes, they are large foundation schools!) – Wales, for instance, allows you to rank your hospital and jobs for FY2 after you have started FY1.

12.1.6 Some things to consider when ranking rotations

- If you are interested in pursuing a career in a particular specialty, completing a 4-month rotation in the job will be a great way of seeing if it is the right specialty for you. A large component of this is seeing how the registrars and consultants work on a regular basis and deciding if the job will make you happy.

- If you would like to free up some spare time to revise for an exam or to build your CV, you should **consider tracks that contain supernumerary rotations**. These are rotations in which you have fewer on-call commitments. However, it is worth noting that these rotations often pay less.

- **Teaching hospitals vs. district generals.** Generally speaking, the advantages of large teaching hospitals are: more on-site specialties, more complex patients, easier access to medical students (if starting a teaching programme), easier access to research, larger cohort of foundation doctors to socialise with, and they tend to be closer to cities and transport links. Whereas, the advantages of district general hospitals are: the staff become a close community, it may take less time to settle in, foundation doctors are able to take on more responsibility and learn hands-on skills, e.g. chest drains, lumbar punctures, etc., and the surrounding accommodation is cheaper.

- **Be careful when using Oriel to rank your tracks.** You will notice the process involves dragging tracks from one side of the webpage across to the other. There have been cases where a less desirable track jumps to the top of the preference list accidentally after it has been dragged across. Triple-check your list of preferences to avoid disappointment.

12.2 Academic foundation programme

In addition to applying for the standard UK Foundation Programme, final year medical students can also apply for the AFP. AFP allows foundation doctors to have protected time for completing academic activities. These academic activities can be focused on one of many varying themes, such as: research, teaching, leadership/ management, and QI. Most AFPs will provide this protected time as part of a 4-month academic placement during FY2, but some

AFPs will spread the protected time over the course of FY1 and FY2. The structure will depend on the foundation school that provides the AFP. A local university is usually responsible for the coordination of any academic placement, which entitles AFP doctors to a wealth of academic resources and provides a great opportunity for teaching medical students.

Typically, AFP doctors will be expected to complete a self-designed project during their academic placement. This should align with the theme of their AFP; for example, completing a study as part of a research themed AFP. This provides a fantastic opportunity for AFP doctors to improve their CV and this could be beneficial for specialty job applications further down the line. It is worth investigating the amount of funding that each foundation school allocates to its AFP doctors. This funding can be very useful for completing projects and presenting findings at conferences. All AFP doctors are allocated to an academic supervisor who will be able to guide these projects, act as a mentor for ongoing development, and facilitate career progression.

The AFP application process involves providing all of the same details as those in the standard UK Foundation Programme application. It also involves an additional section in which applicants must describe their academic achievements to date, i.e. everything that has been covered in *Chapters 5–10*. This provides candidates with an opportunity to demonstrate their affinity towards a particular AFP theme. There are a total of approximately 540 AFP positions across the UK. These positions are provided by 15 Academic Unit of Application(s) (AUoAs). An AUoA is a group of one or more foundation schools that have joined together for the purposes of processing AFP applications. The full list of AUoAs can be found on the foundation programme website:

✐ **www.foundationprogramme.nhs.uk/programmes/2-year-foundation-programme/academic-training**. Each candidate is able to apply to a maximum of two AUoAs, within which they must rank all of the available positions.

> ✏ Always have a plan

Competition is high and applicants must strive towards building their CV during the early years of medical school to give themselves the maximum chance. Once the application deadline has passed, some applicants will be asked to attend an interview. The performance of each candidate at interview will then be considered in combination with their CV and written application to determine if they are successful. Applicants who are unsuccessful automatically become a part of the standard UK Foundation Programme. If this is the case, or if you have already missed the boat for AFP, do not be disheartened. There will still be opportunities for academic training programmes as you progress through your career (see *Section 14.5*).

> **Note:** *The AFP application process is always evolving and so we suggest you refer to the UKFPO website for the latest information ✈ (www.foundationprogramme.nhs.uk).*

12.3 Foundation priority programme

Foundation schools are able to nominate tracks that involve typically less desirable locations and rotations. These tracks will be recruited to in advance of the standard UK Foundation Programme allocation to foundation schools. Applicants are invited to preference the FPPs nominated by each foundation school. Offers are made according to FPAS points (higher scoring applicants will be allocated tracks ahead of lower scoring applicants) and will be made prior to the standard UK Foundation Programme allocation to foundation school places. Applicants who accept an offer for FPP will not be included in the standard UK Foundation Programme allocation. Unsuccessful FPP applicants, or those who decline offers, will automatically be included in the standard UK Foundation Programme allocation to foundation school process. To draw you in, FPPs offer various opportunities, such as:

- Longer foundation training (up to 3 years), which includes freedom to pursue additional training, flexible working, and geographic stability
- Simultaneous management and leadership programmes
- Exposure to academic medicine
- Teaching roles
- Financial support.

12.4 Psychiatry foundation fellowship programme

The PFF Programme has been designed to improve accessibility to psychiatry. Those with a keen interest in psychiatry are encouraged to submit a separate application to the Royal College of Psychiatrists. The application form will be available on the Royal College website (✈ www.rcpsych.ac.uk) from December to January and will evaluate each applicant's commitment to the specialty and understanding of mental health. Using criteria set out by the Royal College, each application will be given a score to determine the overall ranking of applicants. As part of the standard UK Foundation Programme allocation process, you will be allocated to foundation school places in March, and will need to rank the tracks available within your allocated foundation school. Allocations to PFFs will be based on your score determined by the Royal College and your preference order of available PFFs within your allocated foundation school. The UK Foundation Programme Office will identify applicants who are successful in their application to the Royal College and will pre-allocate them a PFF before the allocation of standard UK Foundation Programme tracks.

Note: *Following the release of the standard UK Foundation Programme allocation to foundation school results, applicants who have applied for PFF will have the option to opt out of the selection process for PFF. Applicants who wish to do so, for whatever reason, should email helpdesk@foundationprogramme.nhs.uk within 1 week of being allocated to a foundation school. Opting out of the selection process for PFF does not impact your allocation to a standard UK Foundation Programme track.*

Successful PFF applicants will be supported throughout the 2-year duration of the programme and into Core Psychiatry Training. This support includes funding to access educational opportunities relevant to psychiatry. The aim is to promote interest in psychiatry across the 2-year period, including during non-psychiatric rotations.

Note: *England and Wales will be using the process as described above, Scotland will include PFF posts as part of the FPP allocation process, and Northern Ireland have opted out. Currently, there are approximately 40 PFFs available across 15 foundation schools. No PFFs are available in London.*

For further information regarding PFF benefits and number of PFFs available visit: ➤ www.rcpsych.ac.uk/become-a-psychiatrist/med-students/awards-prizes-and-bursaries/psychiatry-foundation-fellowship.

12.5 Top tips for medical students

- **Be as thorough as you possibly can** when submitting evidence and ranking preferences on Oriel. You have to submit all of your evidence on Oriel as one single document. If you make a mistake there is no going back.

- **Ensure you check all of the important deadlines thoroughly.** There are applicants who have missed out on their preferred location or rotations when they had the required points simply because they had not submitted their preferences on time!

- **Spend time repeating the SJT past papers** on the foundation programme website. There is no need to spend lots of money on many different courses (one is enough). Do not over-stress about this exam.

- **Think long and hard about where you want to work for FY1 and FY2.** It is a great chance to spread your wings and seek out new opportunities.

- **The AFP is a tremendous opportunity to build your portfolio** for future job applications. There are no drawbacks in applying. AFP doctors will still receive at least baseline salary during their academic placement. Unsuccessful applicants automatically become a part of the standard UK Foundation Programme without any consequences.

- **Investigate all of the different AFPs that are available.** Make sure you know exactly what you are applying for and what is expected of you.

- **If the FPP or PFF is aligned to your career goals, you should apply.** Both programmes provide opportunities to opt out and re-join the standard UK Foundation Programme.

> **HOMEWORK 12:**
>
> Reach out to final year medical students or junior doctors who have successfully navigated through the AFP application process. Tell them you are considering applying for the AFP in the future and ask them for their best pieces of advice.

📢 Don't ask, don't get

CHAPTER 13

Taking a FY3

After finishing the foundation programme (FY1 and FY2) many doctors decide to delay the process of entering into specialty training by one year. This is known as taking a FY3. There are many reasons why doctors choose to take a FY3. Common examples include:
- To work *ad hoc* and go travelling for long periods
- To gain experience of working in another country
- To gain experience of working in specialties before applying to them
- To build their CV for specialty applications
- To take a career break for personal reasons.

☼ **Avoid burnout**

It is becoming more common for junior doctors to opt for a FY3. In terms of improving your CV, there is no right or wrong decision here. Junior doctors should base their decision on what they would enjoy most. If you would prefer to progress straight into specialty training, do not fear that you will be disadvantaged. You may not have a lot to gain from taking a FY3 and submitting an application for specialty training during FY2 will somewhat demonstrate your commitment. If you would prefer to take a FY3, there are many options for you to be excited about. However, at the time of applying for specialty training, recruiters might expect you to have more on your CV and will want to know how you spent your FY3. This is even more pertinent to those who decide to take a FY4 and FY5. In this chapter we will cover the most important information about taking a FY3. Our aim is to inspire you with some of the exciting options you have, provide you with a solid understanding of FY3 logistics, and make you aware of the potential pitfalls.

13.1 FY3 clinical roles

Here, we will outline the most popular clinical roles for FY3 doctors. It is important to remember these roles are also available in countries outside of the UK. If you wish to read more about working abroad, see *Chapter 17*. It is also worth bearing in mind that these are examples of paid roles only. There are many voluntary organisations that doctors are able to contribute towards during their FY3. Doctors may also regard FY3 as an opportunity to complete a postgraduate degree.

13.1.1 Locum doctor

Locum doctors play a vital role in healthcare. They are able to alleviate workforce pressures that arise when doctors take leave and when demand for healthcare rises. Essentially, they are an extra pair of hands when called upon. As a locum doctor you are only expected to work on the days that you agree to. This flexibility is one of the big attractions for FY3 doctors, because it allows them to spend their time freely. Commonly, FY3 doctors will work 2 or 3 days a week. However, it is possible for locum doctors to work as regularly as full-time doctors if they wish. Another big attraction is the pay. Locum doctors are paid an hourly rate that is often significantly higher than rates for doctors in full-time roles. The rate of hourly pay is also negotiable before agreeing to work the shift. There are two routine methods of securing work as a locum doctor.

1. **Registering with a locum agency**. There are many agencies with access to both long-term and short-term locum shifts. These agencies will suggest suitable shifts as they become available and will help you to secure them. Some agencies are also able to assist with delivering necessary training and on-site support, completing GMC revalidation, and arranging travel and accommodation. To register with an agency, you must provide professional information, such as: qualifications, GMC number, employment history, references, occupational health checks, DBS checks and so on. The main drawbacks of agencies are that they work with a restricted number of hospitals, they take a cut from your salary, and they may require a fair amount of admin, i.e. phone calls, messages, emails, and paperwork. However, it is likely they will significantly reduce the amount of time you spend searching for jobs and they will ensure you do not forget to complete any aspects of job applications. This is especially important if planning to work abroad!

> **Note:** *A popular alternative to registering with a locum agency is using mobile apps, e.g. Locum's Nest or Patchwork. Using apps like these, locum doctors can secure both long-term and short-term shifts without dealing with an agency. However, this requires you to adopt a more active role in searching for shifts and securing the ones that are suitable. You will still need to complete all of the necessary paperwork that makes you eligible to work in that Trust (unless you are a part of the Trust's bank).*

2. **Applying for a Trust's bank.** Many Trusts anticipate the need for locum doctors and so recruit for 'bank' positions. Being a part of the Trust's bank means that you are willing to be contacted directly by the Trust when locum shifts become available. It also means that you have completed all of the necessary paperwork which ensures you are eligible to work as a locum doctor in that Trust. It is therefore easier to become a part of the bank at a Trust where you have recently worked. Typically, after the bank doctors have been contacted about a shift, they will have the opportunity to secure the shift via a mobile app such as those mentioned above or via email correspondence. Trusts are able to combine their banks so it may be possible for doctors to work for more than one Trust when applying to a singular bank. Doctors can also sign up to multiple Trust banks. The main drawbacks of Trust banks are waiting for an occupational health appointment if you have not worked at the Trust previously, receiving less assistance than those registered with a locum agency, and the shifts have the potential to dry up.

> **Note:** *In 2016, NHS Professionals launched 'Doctors Direct' to provide an alternative method of securing locum shifts. This has become a mixture of the locum agency and Trust bank approaches, with dedicated professionals always available to help, no agency fees, and all profits are re-invested into the NHS. Doctors Direct uses a smart platform, which allows users to view and manage locum bookings via their smartphone:*
> ✈ *www.nhsprofessionals.nhs.uk/DoctorsDirect.*

13.1.2 Junior clinical fellowships/Trust grade posts

These are full-time jobs that are not a part of any formal training route and are a FY2 job equivalent. This means that completing the job successfully during FY3 does not automatically lead you onto the next stage in your training. It also means that you will probably be paid the same as a FY2 doctor and carry similar responsibilities. These jobs may have different names but are most commonly called junior clinical fellowships or Trust grade posts. They are available on either a fixed-term basis (usually 6 or 12 months) or a permanent basis. The nature of the job will depend entirely on the specialty and the employing Trust. They are a brilliant opportunity to gain experience in a particular specialty; some jobs will even provide you with dedicated time to pursue personal interests, such as research (these may be referred to as junior research fellowships). It is crucial to check what the minimum entry requirements are for all Trust grade jobs and fellowships, because many are only available for specialist trainees. Typically, doctors will apply for these positions during their FY2 via online jobsites, e.g. ➤ www.jobs.nhs.uk and ➤ https://apps.trac.jobs.

13.1.3 Undergraduate teaching fellowships

In these roles, junior doctors are employed by an NHS Trust and/or university and are expected to contribute to the design, coordination, and delivery of their undergraduate teaching programmes (including simulation sessions and examinations). Employment can be part-time or full-time and is usually on a 12-month fixed-term basis. Some teaching fellows are supported in gaining formal teaching qualifications, e.g. PGCert in Medical Education. They are also encouraged to participate in research about medical education in their Trust. Typically, there are no clinical commitments. However, there are jobs that involve split commitments between teaching and clinical practice (within a specified specialty). It is also commonplace for undergraduate teaching fellows to work locum shifts at their Trust.

13.2 FY3 logistics

Unfortunately, the process of planning a FY3 is not as simple as finding a job and packing your bags. FY3 doctors are effectively stepping off the conveyor-belt of becoming a consultant or a GP. This disruption to training can become detrimental if not coordinated properly. Here, we will cover the key elements that must be considered when planning a FY3.

13.2.1 Timing

The application process for securing a FY3 clinical role takes place during FY2. Doctors should therefore begin investigating their options for FY3 during FY1, as this will minimise the risk of missing application deadlines during early FY2. Using this same logic, FY3 doctors should begin investigating their year after FY3 during FY2. If your plan involves working abroad or going travelling for long periods during FY3, it is paramount to remember that specialty applications may depend on your ability to access reliable internet and to attend interviews in person. Investigate application timelines thoroughly and make sure that you do not hinder yourself.

13.2.2 Finances

There are some points for FY3 doctors to be aware of specifically. For example, whilst working as a FY3 doctor you will not automatically qualify for maternity leave, sick pay, or pension contributions. Furthermore, you might not have access to study budget money (that you had access to in FY2) when paying for expensive courses and exams. If you intend to go travelling or wish to work abroad, there are also hidden costs, such as visas, vaccinations, security checks, and health checks. You should contact your medical defence organisation to receive help with arranging medical indemnity cover. If they are unable to extend your agreement to include your destination, this can also become an additional cost. Attempt to unearth all of the hidden costs of a FY3; if you are organised and do this in advance you will be able to formulate strategies for saving money.

> **You can never be too organised**

13.2.3 GMC registration and licence to practise

To legally provide medical services in the UK, doctors must have a valid GMC registration and licence to practise. GMC registration is available to those who have achieved the necessary qualifications to practise medicine in the UK. To maintain a valid licence to practise, doctors must collect supporting information about their medical practice and have an annual appraisal conducted by an appropriately trained appraiser. For doctors in training, these requirements are fulfilled by completion of e-portfolio and Annual Reviews of Competence Progression (ARCP). In addition to these requirements, doctors must revalidate every 5 years to show they are up to date and fit to practise. Revalidation can be performed in three ways:

1. **Connection to a designated body and responsible officer.**
   It is the duty of the responsible officer to make a recommendation to the GMC, which indicates if the doctor in question is fit to practise and qualifies for revalidation.

2. **Connection to an approved suitable person.** If a doctor does not have a designated body and responsible officer, it may be possible for them to identify a suitable person (licensed doctor) who can make a recommendation to the GMC. This suitable person must first be approved by the GMC before making any recommendations.
3. **Completing an annual return and revalidation assessment.** If a doctor does not have a responsible officer or an approved suitable person to make a recommendation to the GMC, they must submit an annual return (i.e. employment history) via their GMC Online account. In addition, the doctor must complete a revalidation assessment, which is a 120-question multiple-choice test to be completed within 2 hours.

As a FY3 working in the UK, you will still need to collect supporting information about your medical practice and have an annual appraisal conducted by an appropriately trained appraiser. Note that your Foundation Programme Certificate of Completion (FPCC) awarded at end of FY2 is valid for 3.5 years. Therefore, if you decide to take multiple years out of training, you will need an alternative (Certificate of Readiness to Enter Specialty Training) before applying to specialty jobs. In this instance, it is also important to determine your preferred method for completing revalidation. If you wish to work abroad for FY3, it is possible to keep your GMC registration and relinquish your licence to practise (see *Chapter 17* for more details).

13.3 FY3 pitfalls

- **Don't get too much experience.** If you have decided to do a junior clinical fellowship in a specialty that you wish to pursue as a career, do not breach the upper limit of allowable experience in that specialty before applying for a training job. Many specialties enforce a specific number of months as their upper limit (this excludes experience gained during FY1 and FY2), e.g.:
  - surgery – 18 months
  - anaesthetics – 18 months
  - obstetrics and gynaecology – 24 months

  Check the most recent person specifications for training jobs in your desired specialty.

- **Do not become deskilled**. The next stage in your career after FY3 may be very challenging and so it is important to prepare for what lies ahead. If you decide to take a significant break from clinical practice, enquire about Health Education England's Supported Return to Training schemes (SuppoRTT). They can provide enhanced supervision, refresher courses, mentoring, workshops, and funding for doctors who are looking to re-enter the workplace safely.

- **Do not waste it**. Do your best to achieve something during your FY3. Dedicate time to activities that you are truly passionate about and make lasting memories.

> **Note:** *FY3 is not the only opportunity to take time out of training. Although uncommon, it is possible for students to take a sabbatical year during medical school. It is important to ask your clinical sub-deans for guidance if you wish for this to happen. A more common alternative is to take time out during higher specialty training. UK doctors in higher specialty training can take time out of programme for approved clinical training (OOPT) or time out of programme for clinical experience (OOPE). The crucial difference here is that OOPT can count towards your specialty training (taking you closer to becoming a consultant or GP), whereas OOPE cannot. Both OOPT and OOPE must be agreed long in advance of departure by contacting the relevant regional postgraduate dean, training programme director, Royal College and the GMC. There are also recognised options for higher specialty trainees to take time out of programme for research and time out of programme for a career break, e.g. to work in industry, fulfil domestic responsibilities and ill health. If you wish to read more about taking time out of training, visit: ◄ www.nottingham.ac.uk/careers/students/graduatejobs/typesofjobs/medicine/time-out.aspx.*

13.4 Top tips for medical students

- **FY3 is a great opportunity to make your CV stand out from the crowd**. Be organised and secure a position that will catch the recruiter's eye.

- **Remember, you can apply to multiple positions simultaneously.** See what offers you get before making any big decisions.

- **You should start considering your options for FY3 during FY1.** That way you can begin to prepare yourself for the application process, which will take place during FY2. Preparing for FY3 any sooner than FY1 is unlikely to be of any benefit.

- **If you know any FY2 doctors, ask them for information about FY3.** They will be well informed about all of the different options.

13.5 Advice from the experts

Professor Chloe Orkin:

"I went to Botswana as an OOPE as part of a government and third sector collaboration to set up the first anti-retroviral treatment programme for the north of Botswana. It was the best thing I ever did, and the hardest. I worked 13-hour days from a portacabin with no mobile phone for several months. I had no TV, no sofa and no landline, but it was the most rewarding job I have ever done, and I had the ability to do it with my partner who is a nurse."

Mr Gareth Dobson:

"On completing Foundation Training I had planned to work abroad for a year. My aim was to work within a large trauma centre or A&E, hoping this would support my application to neurosurgical training the following year. Unfortunately, I was unsuccessful in obtaining a post in any of the large centres I applied for. Despite offers from other smaller centres abroad, I decided to stay put and I organised a stand-alone post as a neurosurgical SHO for 1 year. Whilst this post undoubtedly provided me with invaluable knowledge, skills and experience which supported my application to training, I do regret not taking the opportunity to work abroad."

Dr Jeeves Wijesuriya:

"I took a sabbatical year during medical school to be president of my Student Union and the United Hospitals Med Group for medical schools across London. This gave me loads of leadership and management experience (as well as another year at medical school!). I also did a BSc in Medical Education alongside this which gave me a really solid academic grounding, which helped me later in my career."

Dr Harrison Carter:

"I took a year away from clinical medicine to be an NHS England and Improvement National Medical Director's Clinical Fellow. I was working for the COVID-19 national strategic incident director in the Emergency Preparedness, Resilience and Response team. My day-to-day role was in a very high-level position in the Incident Director's private office working on the NHS's response to COVID-19 in England and the end of the transition period for EU exit. I also worked on restoring services to tackle waiting lists and other winter pressures projects. My reports and work were being read by senior government officials, No. 10 Downing Street and the Cabinet Office on a weekly basis. I was engaging with Royal College presidents and supporting decisions that were central to the NHS's ability to function safely for patients. I also worked as part of the national incident coordination centre. It was an absolute privilege to be in this position. It was hugely beneficial to understand the inner workings of government and parliament as well as to appreciate the difficulties associated with working nationally to ensure the NHS can deliver for patients and protect staff. The job was all-consuming and all-encompassing."

HOMEWORK 13:

When you reach FY1, begin to investigate your options for FY3. If you might work as a locum in the same area where you are currently working, ask your rota coordinators if you can be a part of the Trust bank.

Always have a plan

CHAPTER 14

NHS training routes

After completing the foundation programme, the next step for junior doctors in their training is to enter into core (internal) medicine training (IMT), core surgical training (CST), acute care common stem (ACCS), or a run-through training programme. This of course depends on what specialty you wish to pursue. In this chapter, we will explain each of these training pathways in detail and discuss the most important factors to consider. We will also explain the ways of entering academic training posts which allow doctors to combine their specialty training with research or education training.

14.1 Core (internal) medicine training and higher specialty training

The IMT programme involves rotating across a range of medical specialties. These specialties will vary from trainee to trainee. However, all internal medicine trainees will gain experience in intensive care medicine, geriatric medicine and outpatients. IMT lasts for 2 or 3 years, depending on the higher specialty training programme that follows. If the higher specialty training programme is in 'group 1', IMT will last for 3 years (see *Figure 14.1*). If the higher specialty training programme is in 'group 2', IMT will last for 2 years (see *Figure 14.2*). Entry into IMT does not guarantee you any form of higher specialty training programme. Instead, trainees compete with one another for positions in higher specialty training programmes. Some specialties are more competitive than others and it is always worth looking online for the competition ratios (applicants : positions) to see how contested the entry is into your desired specialty (see *Section 14.5*). For highly competitive specialties in particular, this creates a bottleneck, which can be extremely frustrating for trainees and causes some unsuccessful applicants to take time out of training or pursue less competitive medical specialties.

Figure 14.1: The physician training pathway – Group 1 specialties (dual Certificate of Completion of Training (CCT)). KBA – Knowledge-Based Assessment; SCE – Specialty Certificate Examination.

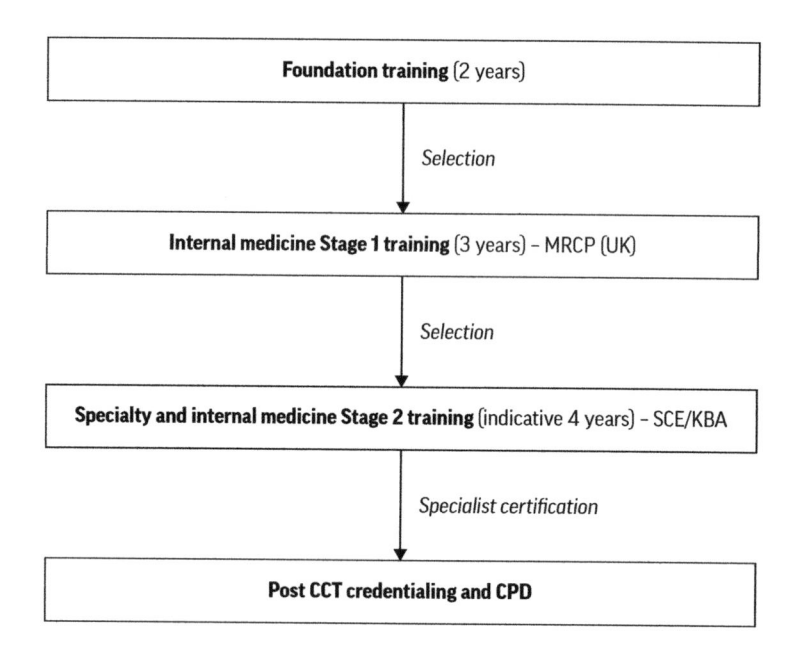

```
┌─────────────────────────────────────────────────────────────┐
│              Foundation training (2 years)                   │
└─────────────────────────────────────────────────────────────┘
                            │ Selection
                            ▼
┌─────────────────────────────────────────────────────────────┐
│      Internal medicine Stage 1 training (3 years) – MRCP (UK)│
└─────────────────────────────────────────────────────────────┘
                            │ Selection
                            ▼
┌─────────────────────────────────────────────────────────────┐
│ Specialty and internal medicine Stage 2 training (indicative 4 years) – SCE/KBA │
└─────────────────────────────────────────────────────────────┘
                            │ Specialist certification
                            ▼
┌─────────────────────────────────────────────────────────────┐
│              Post CCT credentialing and CPD                  │
└─────────────────────────────────────────────────────────────┘
```

Group 1 specialties: acute internal medicine, cardiology, clinical pharmacology and therapeutics, endocrinology and diabetes mellitus, gastroenterology, genitourinary medicine, geriatric medicine, infectious diseases (except when dual with medical microbiology or virology), neurology, palliative medicine, renal medicine, respiratory medicine, and rheumatology.

Figure 14.2: The physician training pathway – Group 2 specialties (dual CCT). KBA – Knowledge-Based Assessment; SCE – Specialty Certificate Examination.

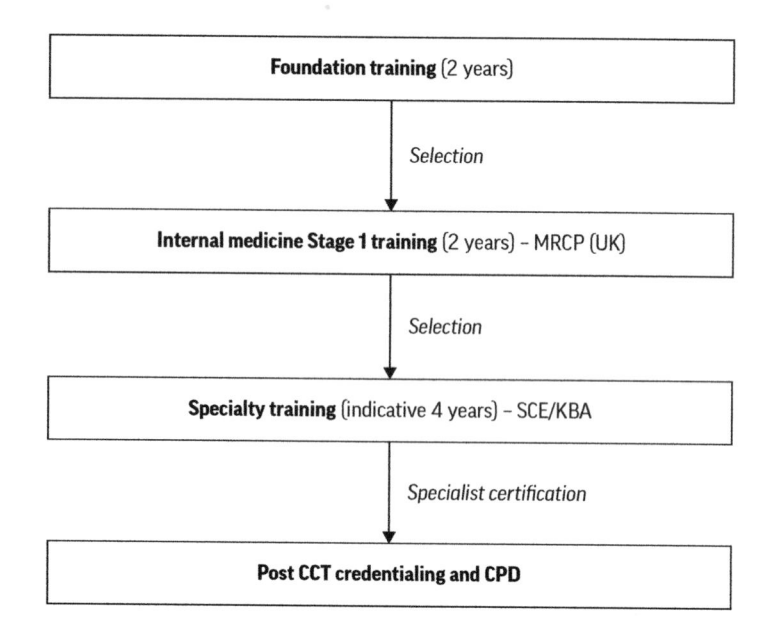

```
┌─────────────────────────────────────────────────────────────┐
│              Foundation training (2 years)                   │
└─────────────────────────────────────────────────────────────┘
                            │ Selection
                            ▼
┌─────────────────────────────────────────────────────────────┐
│      Internal medicine Stage 1 training (2 years) – MRCP (UK)│
└─────────────────────────────────────────────────────────────┘
                            │ Selection
                            ▼
┌─────────────────────────────────────────────────────────────┐
│      Specialty training (indicative 4 years) – SCE/KBA       │
└─────────────────────────────────────────────────────────────┘
                            │ Specialist certification
                            ▼
┌─────────────────────────────────────────────────────────────┐
│              Post CCT credentialing and CPD                  │
└─────────────────────────────────────────────────────────────┘
```

Group 2 specialties: allergy, audiovestibular medicine, aviation and space medicine, clinical genetics, clinical neurophysiology, dermatology, haematology, immunology, infectious diseases (when dual with medical microbiology or virology), medical oncology, medical ophthalmology, nuclear medicine, paediatric cardiology, pharmaceutical medicine, rehabilitation medicine and sport and exercise medicine. Clinical oncology, medical microbiology, medical virology, and occupational medicine will also recruit trainees who have completed the first two years of IMT. Trainees will also be able to apply for intensive care medicine single CCT training after 2 years of IMT.

14.2 Core surgical training and higher specialty training

The CST programme involves rotating across a range of surgical specialties (see *Figures 14.3–14.5*). These may be themed towards one particular specialty or sub-specialty. Core surgical training lasts for 2 years. Like IMT, entry into CST does not guarantee you any form of higher specialty training programme. Instead, core surgical trainees compete with one another for positions in higher specialty training programmes. Again, some specialties are more competitive than others and it is always worth looking online for the competition ratios (applicants : positions) to see how contested the entry is into your desired specialty (see *Section 14.5*). Again, for highly competitive specialties in particular, this creates a bottleneck which can be extremely frustrating for trainees and causes some unsuccessful applicants to take time out of training or pursue less competitive surgical specialties.

14.3 Run-through training programmes

Run-through training programmes provide an opportunity for doctors to enter higher specialty training directly (and become a ST1). The duration of the training programme depends on the specialty. For general practice (GP), training lasts 3 years. For other specialties, training lasts between 5 and 7 years. After a doctor has completed their run-through training programme, they are able to become a qualified GP or a consultant in their specialty. There is only one application process at the beginning of the programme. Thereafter, doctors are recruited for the entire duration of their training.

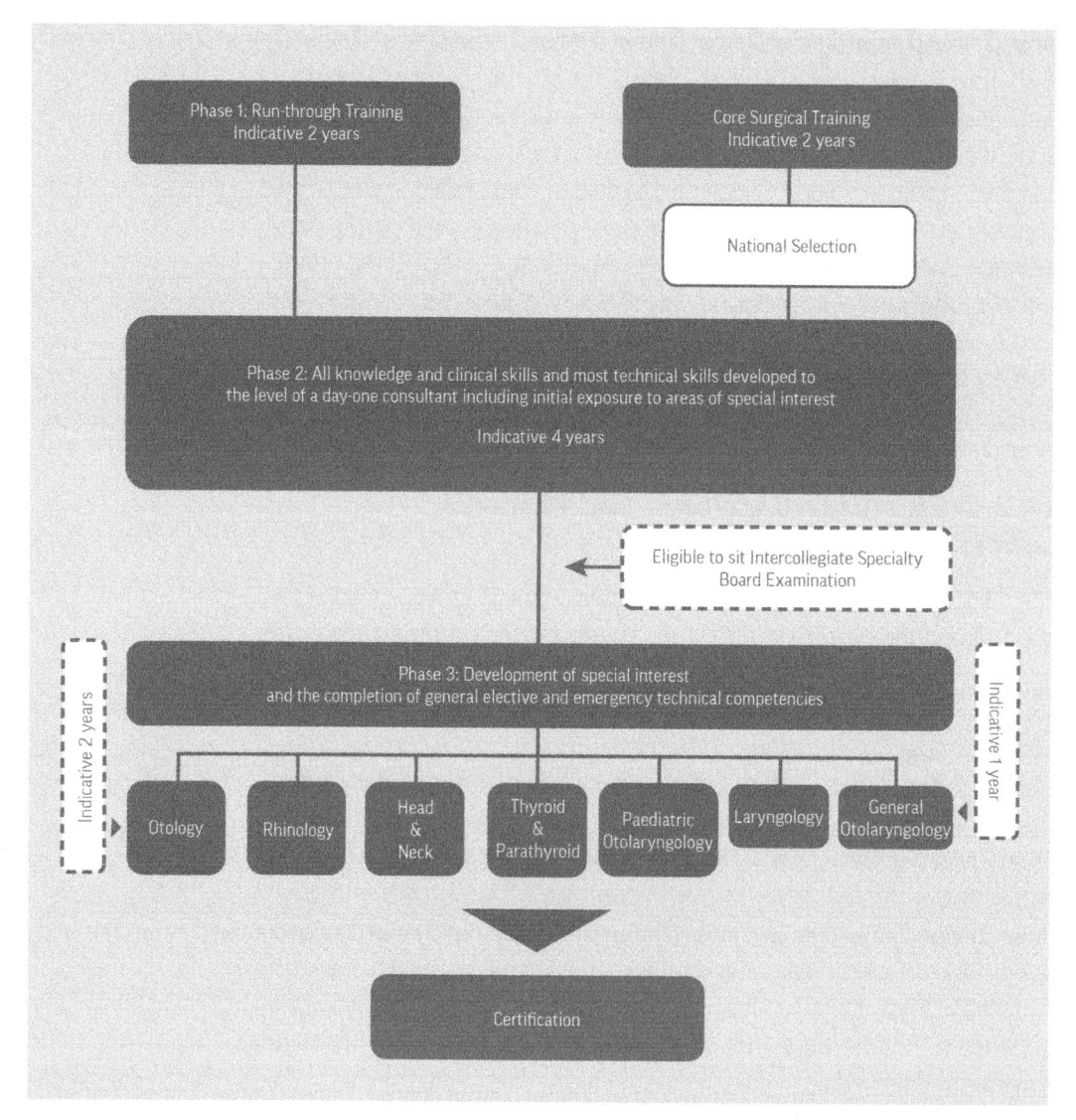

Figure 14.3: Training pathway for otolaryngology. Surgical specialties that follow a very similar training path to otolaryngology include: vascular, cardiothoracic, oral and maxillofacial, paediatric, plastic, trauma and orthopaedics, and urology. However, for the most up-to-date training information that is specific to each surgical specialty, see **www.iscp.ac.uk/iscp/curriculum-2021/**. Reproduced from the Joint Committee on Surgical Training (JCST): *Intercollegiate Surgical Curriculum Programme (ISCP)* at **www.iscp.ac.uk**.

Foundation doctors often regard this as an attractive method of training. Consequently, the competition ratios for run-through training programmes are frequently high. This creates a bottleneck and forces many unsuccessful applicants to take FY3s or to pursue less

NHS TRAINING ROUTES

CHAPTER 14

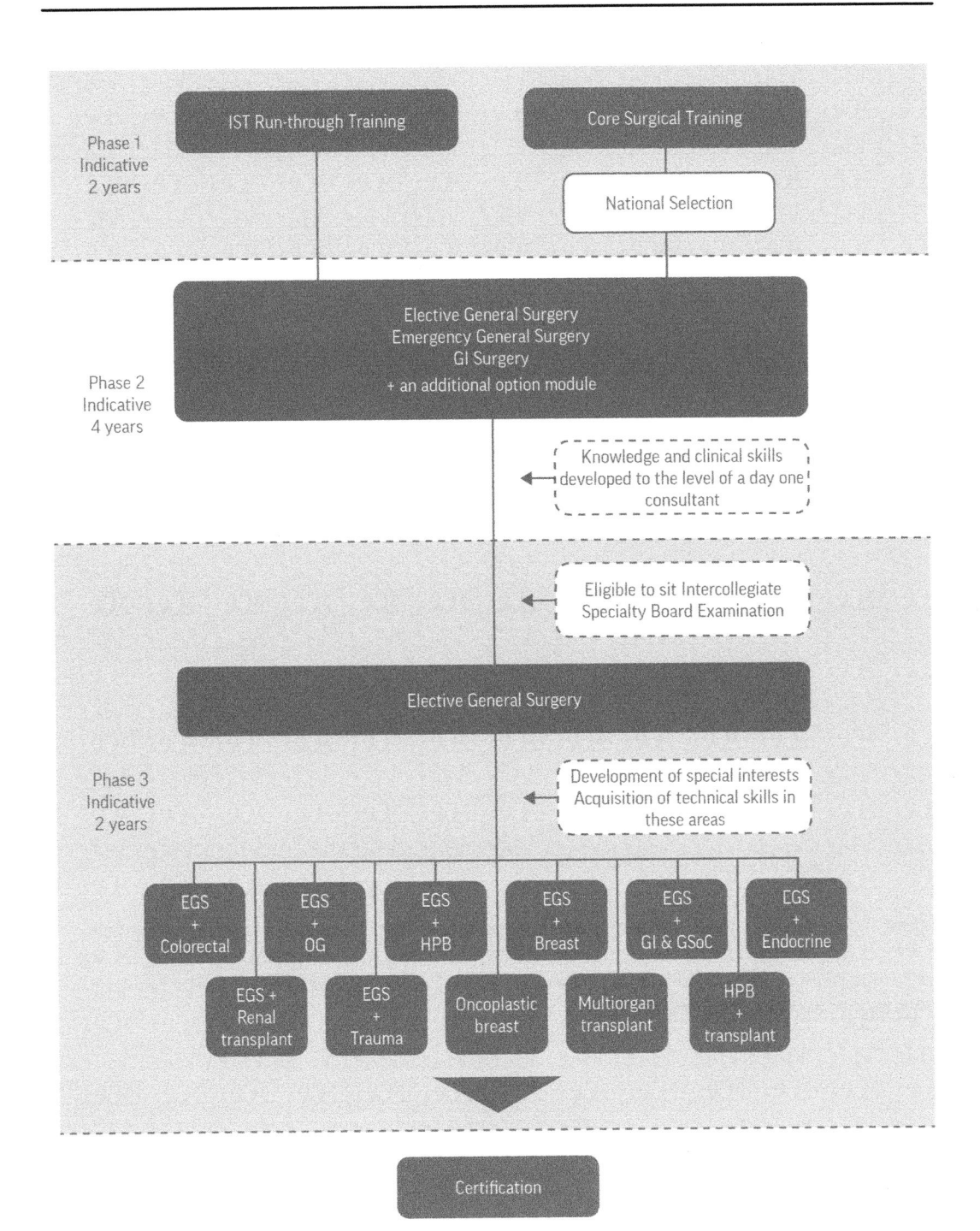

Figure 14.4: Training pathway for general surgery. Reproduced from the Joint Committee on Surgical Training (JCST): *Intercollegiate Surgical Curriculum Programme (ISCP)* at **www.iscp.ac.uk**. If you would like to read more about surgical training curricula, the most up-to-date information can be found at: **www.iscp.ac.uk/iscp/curriculum-2021/**.

```
Phase 1: Clinical Neuroscience Skills, Common Surgical Core and Emergency Medicine
including Neurosurgery and a selection of Neuroradiology, Neuro Intensive Care, Neurology,
Neuropathology, Emergency Medicine and a ralated surgical specialty

Indicative 2 years
```

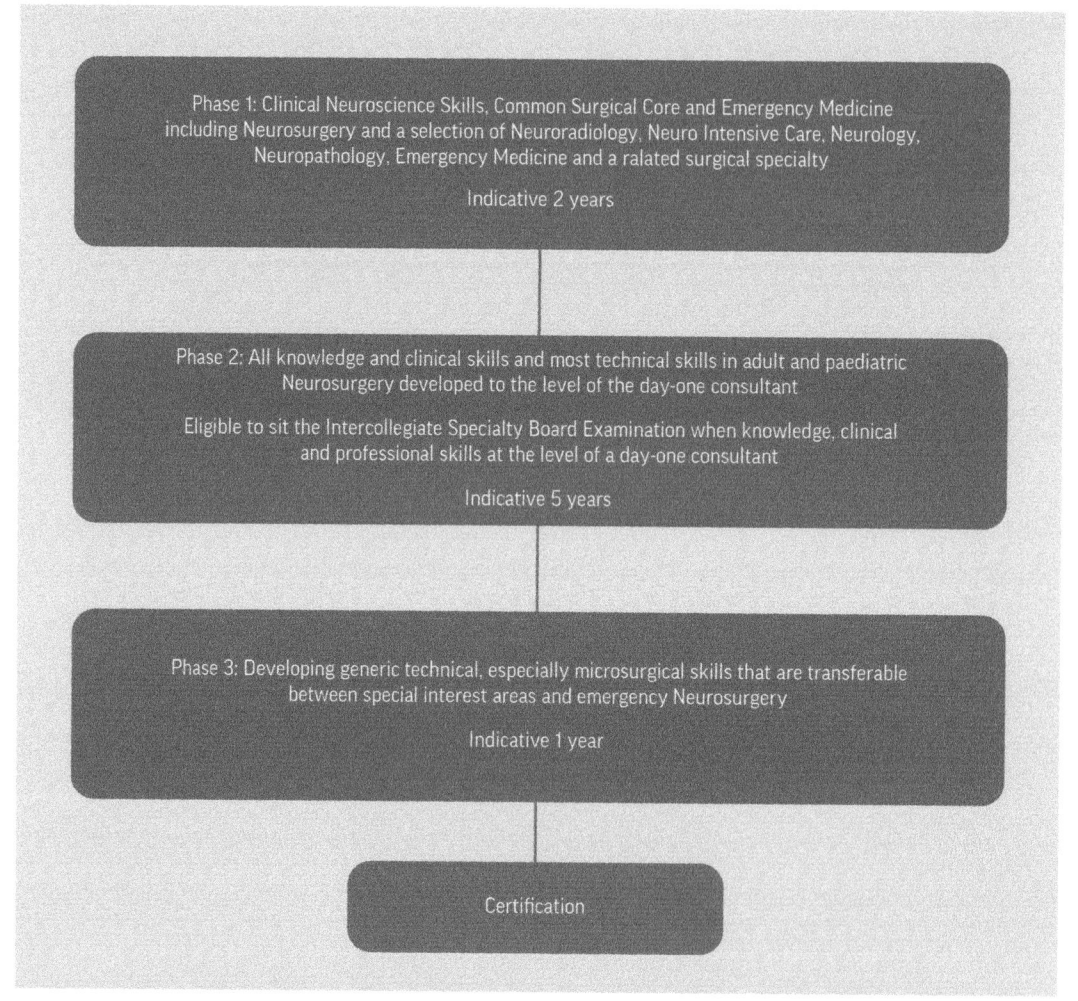

```
Phase 2: All knowledge and clinical skills and most technical skills in adult and paediatric
Neurosurgery developed to the level of the day-one consultant

Eligible to sit the Intercollegiate Specialty Board Examination when knowledge, clinical
and professional skills at the level of a day-one consultant

Indicative 5 years
```

```
Phase 3: Developing generic technical, especially microsurgical skills that are transferable
between special interest areas and emergency Neurosurgery

Indicative 1 year
```

```
Certification
```

Figure 14.5: Training pathway for neurosurgery. Reproduced from the Joint Committee on Surgical Training (JCST): *Intercollegiate Surgical Curriculum Programme (ISCP)* at **www.iscp.ac.uk**. If you would like to read more about surgical training curricula, the most up-to-date information can be found at: **www.iscp.ac.uk/iscp/curriculum-2021/**.

competitive training programmes. Examples of specialties that offer run-through training programmes include paediatrics, obstetrics and gynaecology, ophthalmology, radiology, cardiothoracic surgery, and neurosurgery.

14.4 Acute care common stem

ACCS is a 3 year programme that involves rotating through acute medical specialties. Years 1 and 2 of the programme involve rotating through emergency medicine, acute internal medicine, anaesthetics, and intensive care medicine. The third year of the programme is tailored to the trainee and the higher specialty training they wish to pursue (also known as their parent specialty). ACCS is the only training programme that allows doctors to enter higher specialty training in emergency medicine. It is also a popular alternative training programme that allows doctors to enter higher specialty training in general internal medicine, acute internal medicine, anaesthesia, or intensive care medicine. Recruitment for ACCS is performed by the parent specialty. Therefore, before your application begins, it is important to determine which acute medical specialty you wish to pursue so that you are able to prepare a suitable portfolio. The membership examinations that ACCS trainees must pass to progress into higher specialty training depend on the parent specialty. Hence, it is not necessary for foundation doctors to complete membership examinations before entering ACCS. Like IMT and CST, entry into ACCS does not guarantee you any form of higher specialty training programme. Instead, ACCS trainees compete with one another for positions in higher specialty training programmes. Again, some specialties are more competitive than others and the competition ratios (applicants : positions) will determine the severity of the bottleneck.

14.5 Competition ratios

The competition ratios for specialty training in 2020 can be found in *Table 14.1* (which represents round 1 of applications) and *Table 14.2* (which represents round 2 of applications). The key differences between round 1 and round 2 are the entry and the timescale. Round 1 is mostly for CT1/ST1 entry and begins in November, whereas round 2 is mostly for ST3 entry and begins in July. It is possible to apply for round 1 and round 2, in which case your application in round 1 will have no effect on your round 2 application (and vice versa).

Table 14.1: Competition ratios 2020 – round 1

Specialty	Entry level	UK Applications	Posts	Ratio
ACCS anaesthetics/core anaesthetics	CT1/ST1	1479	569	2.60
ACCS emergency medicine	CT1/ST1	863	348	2.48
Broad based training	CT1/ST1	109	13	8.38
Cardiothoracic surgery	CT1/ST1	129	13	9.92
Clinical radiology	CT1/ST1	1308	311	4.21
Community sexual and reproductive health	CT1/ST1	108	6	18.00
Core psychiatry training	CT1/ST1	895	410	2.18
Core surgical training	CT1/ST1	2322	605	3.84
General practice	CT1/ST1	5770	3836	1.50
Histopathology	CT1/ST1	261	97	2.69
Internal medicine training	CT1/ST1	2798	1610	1.74
Neurosurgery	CT1/ST1	220	26	8.46
Obstetrics and gynaecology	CT1/ST1	672	256	2.63
Ophthalmology	CT1/ST1	430	75	5.73
Oral and maxillofacial surgery	CT1/ST1	32	10	3.20
Paediatrics	CT1/ST1	712	461	1.54
Public health medicine	CT1/ST1	933	77	12.12
Trauma and orthopaedic surgery (Scotland only)	CT1/ST1	221	9	24.56
Cardiothoracic surgery	ST3	41	7	5.86
Neurosurgery	ST3	22	1	22.00
Ophthalmology	ST3	65	22	2.95
Oral and maxillofacial surgery	ST3	16	23	0.70

Reproduced from https://specialtytraining.hee.nhs.uk/Competition-Ratios under the Open Government Licence v3.0.

NHS TRAINING ROUTES   CHAPTER 14

Table 14.2: Competition ratios 2020 – round 2

Specialty	Entry level	UK Applications	Posts	Ratio
Acute internal medicine	ST3	510	94	5.43
Allergy	ST3	11	3	3.67
Anaesthetics	ST3	758	353	2.15
Audiovestibular medicine	ST3	9	6	1.50
Cardiology	ST3	533	131	4.07
Clinical genetics	ST3	40	13	3.08
Clinical neurophysiology	ST3	31	10	3.10
Clinical oncology	ST3	170	49	3.47
Clinical pharmacology and therapeutics	ST3	12	14	0.86
Combined infection training	ST3	206	54	3.81
Dermatology	ST3	166	42	3.95
Diagnostic neuropathology	ST3	8	4	2.00
Emergency medicine	ST3	141	47	3.00
Endocrinology and diabetes mellitus	ST3	325	74	4.39
Gastroenterology	ST3	373	79	4.72
General and vascular surgery	ST3	574	123	4.67
Genito-urinary medicine	ST3	31	53	0.58
Geriatric medicine	ST3	392	202	1.94
Haematology	ST3	195	73	2.67
Immunology	ST3	20	12	1.67
Intensive care medicine	ST3	430	289	1.49
Medical oncology	ST3	185	39	4.74

(continued)

Table 14.2: *(continued)*

Specialty	Entry level	UK Applications	Posts	Ratio
Medical ophthalmology	ST3	7	3	2.33
Metabolic medicine	ST3	23	12	1.92
Neurology	ST3	207	50	4.14
Occupational medicine	ST3	35	12	2.92
Otolaryngology	ST3	131	23	5.70
Paediatric and perinatal pathology	ST3	7	9	0.78
Paediatric surgery	ST3	50	6	8.33
Paediatrics	ST3	203	45	4.51
Palliative medicine	ST3	137	49	2.80
Plastic surgery	ST3	190	41	4.63
Rehabilitation medicine	ST3	36	27	1.33
Renal medicine	ST3	227	67	3.39
Respiratory medicine	ST3	407	74	5.50
Rheumatology	ST3	199	33	6.03
Sport and exercise medicine	ST3	32	11	2.91
Trauma and orthopaedic surgery	ST3	715	125	5.72
Urology	ST3	146	64	2.28
Child and adolescent psychiatry	ST4	72	56	1.29
Emergency medicine	ST4	103	57	1.81
Forensic psychiatry	ST4	55	34	1.62
Forensic and child/adolescent psychiatry	ST4	4	3	1.33
General psychiatry	ST4	174	155	1.12

(continued)

Table 14.2: *(continued)*

Specialty	Entry level	UK Applications	Posts	Ratio
General psychiatry and forensic psychiatry	ST4	6	2	3.00
General and medical psychotherapy	ST4	35	9	3.89
General psychiatry and old age psychiatry	ST4	79	63	1.25
Medical psychotherapy	ST4	14	4	3.50
Old age psychiatry	ST4	57	60	0.95
Paediatric cardiology	ST4	44	7	6.29
Paediatrics	ST4	173	77	2.25
Psychiatry of learning disability	ST4	22	45	0.49
Psychiatry of learning disability and child/adolescent psychiatry	ST4	8	7	1.14

Reproduced from https://specialtytraining.hee.nhs.uk/Competition-Ratios under the Open Government Licence v3.0.

14.6 Academic training routes

The structure of academic training after FY2 is different within each country in the UK and within each specialty. In the remainder of this chapter, we will explain the structure of academic training that is present in England. For information about academic training in Wales, Scotland or Northern Ireland, please visit the relevant deanery's website:

- https://heiw.nhs.wales/education-and-training/specialty-training/academic-medicine
- www.scotlanddeanery.nhs.scot
- www.nimdta.gov.uk/specialty-training/information-for-specialty-trainees/spec-academic.

In England there are two types of academic training after FY2: the Academic Clinical Fellowship (ACF) and the Clinical Lectureship. It is important to bear in mind that applicants to these programmes are not required to have completed an AFP.

14.6.1 Academic clinical fellowships

These programmes provide doctors with an opportunity to carry out research or education training alongside their clinical commitments. Typically, 25% of a trainee's paid working hours will be protected for non-clinical activities. These hours may be spread out over the duration of the ACF or they may be provided as an academic placement. The non-clinical activities within ACFs vary, as do the entry points; some programmes commence straight after FY2, whilst others begin during higher specialty training. Therefore, if your ACF application is unsuccessful in the first instance, you may still have an opportunity to apply for another ACF in the future. If you are interested in pursuing an ACF post, it is worth visiting the websites of deaneries and reviewing the available programmes. ACFs are usually advertised during the autumn. Successfully completing an ACF gives doctors a great advantage when applying for future jobs. It also puts doctors in a great position to pursue further academia such as an MD or a PhD.

14.6.2 Clinical lectureship

These programmes are for doctors in higher specialty training who have already completed an MD or a PhD. They are designed to allow trainees to complete postdoctoral research alongside their clinical commitments. Their duration can be up to 4 years.

14.7 Top tips for medical students

- If you are interested in a particular specialty, **take a look online at the competition ratios** for entry into higher specialty training. This will give you an insight to what you are up against and will probably motivate you to start working on your CV.

- If your desired specialty provides run-through training, **you might have to start working on your CV early**. You will probably be expected to have a comprehensive portfolio for the application process which occurs during FY2.

- It is good to be familiar with the different training routes. However, **these will change over time**. Do not worry about them too much whilst you are at medical school but make sure you are aware of the most up-to-date training pathways when you become a junior doctor.

CHAPTER 15

General practice

General practice remains the commonest training pathway for doctors in the UK. It is therefore important for medical students to be aware of the recruitment process and career prospects that are specific to general practice. Unlike the typical portfolio–interview selection process, entry to GP training is determined by a candidate's Single Transferable Score (STS), which is calculated according to their performance in:
- the Multi-Specialty Recruitment Assessment (MSRA)
- a selection centre face-to-face assessment.

The STS allows each candidate to be considered for all GP entry level (GPST1) jobs across the UK. Preference is given in order of STS.

15.1 Multi-Specialty Recruitment Assessment

The MSRA is a computer-based assessment and is used by many specialties to score candidates who apply for entry level training jobs. These specialties include general practice, obstetrics and gynaecology, psychiatry (core and CAMHS), radiology, ophthalmology, community and sexual reproductive health, and neurosurgery. The MSRA consists of two papers: Professional Dilemmas and Clinical Problem-Solving.

15.1.1 Professional dilemmas paper (40% of overall STS)

The theme of this 110-minute paper is similar to the SJT. Candidates are presented with professional dilemmas and their score will depend on how closely their response correlates to GMC professional guidance (*Table 15.1*).

15.1.2 Clinical problem-solving paper (20% of overall STS)

This 75-minute paper is designed to test a candidate's clinical knowledge of general medicine (see *Table 15.2*). The content is aimed at Foundation Programme level and covers 12 areas:
- Cardiovascular

- Dermatology/ENT/ophthalmology
- Endocrinology/metabolic
- Gastroenterology/nutrition
- Infectious disease/haematology/immunology/allergies/genetics
- Musculoskeletal
- Paediatrics
- Pharmacology and therapeutics
- Psychiatry/neurology
- Renal/urology
- Reproductive
- Respiratory.

15.1.3 MSRA scoring

The MSRA scores of all GP candidates are fairly adjusted to provide a mean of 250 with a standard deviation of 40 for each paper. The scores are then split into four bands. Candidates who find themselves in Band 1 will have achieved the lowest scores and will not be able to continue their application. All others will progress to the selection centre face-to-face assessment. A noteworthy exception to this applies to those who achieve a combined score greater than 550 (approximately top 10% of candidates), who qualify for the Direct Pathway to Offers. These candidates are not required to attend the selection centre face-to-face assessment and are more likely to gain their first choice of destination and programme.

Table 15.1: Professional Dilemmas paper scoring

Standardised score range	Approximate % scoring in this range	Score Band	Performance
Below 170	5%	1	Very poor level of performance
171–180	3%	1	
181–210	11%	2	Below average performance
211–230	11%	2	
231–250	16%	3	Good level of performance
251–270	20%	3	
271–290	21%	3	
291–310	11%	4	Very good level of performance
Above 310	3%	4	

Adapted from ➔ https://gprecruitment.hee.nhs.uk.

Table 15.2: Clinical Problem-Solving paper scoring

Standardised score range	Approximate % scoring in this range	Score Band	Performance
Below 170	5%	1	Very poor level of performance
171–180	2%	1	
181–210	10%	2	Below average performance
211–230	12%	2	
231–250	17%	3	Good level of performance
251–270	20%	3	
271–290	20%	3	
291–310	12%	4	Very good level of performance
Above 310	2%	4	

Adapted from ◀ https://gprecruitment.hee.nhs.uk.

> **Note:** *For details on how the MSRA is used for recruitment in specialties other than general practice, please visit the relevant Royal College website.*

15.2 Selection centre face-to-face assessment (40% of overall STS)

The selection centre face-to-face assessment is similar to an OSCE. Candidates spend approximately 3 hours at the selection centre and during this time they must complete separate tasks. The assessors will score candidate performance in communication skills, empathy and sensitivity, conceptual thinking and problem solving, and professional integrity.

> **Note:** *All GPST1 offers are made on the condition of being able to supply three satisfactory references from previous educational or clinical supervisors. Make a good impression with your supervisors during foundation years and contact them early when chasing references!*

15.3 GP specialty training

GPST lasts for a minimum of 3 years. This usually consists of 18 months of hospital rotations, which can include general medicine, old age medicine, paediatrics, obstetrics and gynaecology,

A&E, palliative care, dermatology, ophthalmology, and ENT. Typically, the remaining 18 months is spent working in a GP practice. An increasingly popular alternative is to complete GPST over 4 years as part of an ACF (spending 1 year on academic projects) (see Section 14.6.1) or Global Health Fellowship (spending 1 year working overseas in remote communities). These programmes are specific to Deaneries across the UK and recruitment is separate from the national process outlined above. For more detailed information on Global Health Fellowships, see: ✦ **https://gprecruitment.hee.nhs.uk/recruitment/ghf**.

15.4 Portfolio GP

Unless you apply for a 4-year GP training programme, enhancing your CV at medical school and during foundation years will not necessarily benefit your application to GPST. However, once you become a fully qualified GP, CV enhancement plays a significant role in career progression and variation. Throughout their careers, GPs can enjoy opportunities to adjust their clinical time-commitments and take on multiple roles. GPs who do so are called Portfolio GPs. Roles can include:

- **Becoming a GP with an extended role (GPwER)**, previously known as GP with specialist interest (GPwSI). This involves gaining specialist training or qualifications (often a diploma) and working in specialties outside of the GP setting. Common specialist interests are dermatology, women's health, sports medicine, reproductive health, A&E, cardiology, and COPD. However, there are many more to consider.

- **Becoming a partner of a practice**. This involves becoming a part-owner of a GP practice, managing its operations, and sharing profits that are generated.

- **Taking on a teaching role at a university**.

- **Joining a local medical committee or health board**, e.g. Care Commissioning Group.

- **Contributing to research**.

- **Starting your own business**.

These are just a few examples of how portfolio GPs achieve job variation and career satisfaction. This everlasting flexibility is undoubtedly one of the biggest attractions for those considering a career in general practice.

15.5 Insight from GPs and GP trainees

Case study – GP Registrar

Dr Jeeves Wijesuriya
GP Registrar ST3, Homerton University Hospital
Chair of the BMA UK Junior Doctors Committee (2016–19)
Trustee for Medical Aid Films Charity
Care Quality Commission Special Advisor
Former Academic Foundation Doctor

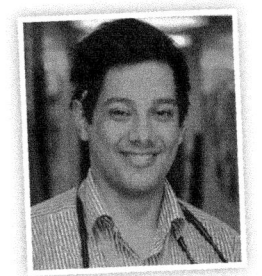

What attracted you to general practice?

I suppose I knew I wanted to be a GP very early on in medical school. I really wanted a career that offered diversity and the opportunity to do lots of different things. General practice work is sessional, which means you can control how much you work and when. Because it is under-recruited for nationally, you have the freedom to work anywhere on your own terms effectively. Often GPs will do medical education work with universities. Many get involved with healthcare organisations like confederations or clinical commissioning groups. There is also the opportunity to be a partner in your practice and run what is akin to a small business. That is just a handful of examples of what you can do!

I really wanted a diverse career and to do different things throughout it alongside clinical work. General practice is one of the few careers that offers you the ability to do that. Whilst I miss working in large teams and the social aspects of that, I certainly don't miss being knackered after the night shifts or the long ward rounds! The other really great thing about general practice is the ability to develop a special interest. Whether that's minor surgery, paediatrics or palliative care, there are so many opportunities to develop a particular interest! I really liked that versatility because I enjoyed so many of my jobs (though certainly not all of them) and knew that in my career I'd want to see different types of patients and cases to keep my career varied and interesting. I also knew I'd then be able to do a bit more of the things I really enjoyed like paediatrics! I also spent some time working reduced hours as a trainee chairing the BMA UK Junior Doctors Committee, where I was able to lead the national negotiation of the UK Junior Doctors Contract with employers and government, helping to bring the longstanding junior doctors' dispute to an end. This experience was tremendous and gave me insights into the healthcare system itself. Working with groups like the GMC and Health Education bodies to improve training systems also gave me a greater appreciation of how training worked. I would really recommend taking up opportunities like these and the chief registrar programmes for example ⯈ (www.rcplondon.ac.uk/projects/chief-registrar-programme), as they really provide great opportunities to see how Trusts and organisations actually work behind the scenes.

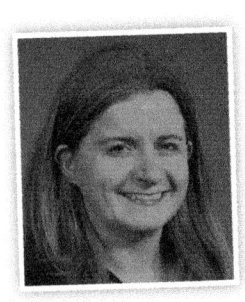

Case study – GP and medical educator

Dr Rachel Holliday MBChB MRCGP PGCertHE

GP in Urgent Care Centre (Countess of Chester Hospital) and Out of Hours GP

Year 3 Director and Community Clinical Tutor, Liverpool Medical School

What attracted you to general practice?

It provides a wide breadth of clinical experience and exposure – the days are never dull!

There is a privilege of continuity with patients and their families. There is also flexibility in career progression; a portfolio career can evolve to incorporate teaching, research, management, and specialty interests. Personally, I have become involved in teaching.

I find it is a privilege to meet and teach the brilliant doctors of tomorrow. Their enthusiasm and curiosity is wonderfully infectious.

What are the drawbacks of general practice?

If I was working as a full-time GP in a practice setting, I would be concerned about the risk of burnout due to the workload.

What is your advice for those considering general practice?

Keep your options open. Choose broad specialties early in your career (A&E, general practice, general medicine) so that you are in a good position to follow the subject that you really enjoy. I find a mixed role (in my case teaching alongside clinical work) is a good way to prevent burnout. Medical careers are long and there are so many exciting opportunities to enjoy along the way – don't be scared to try something new! Be kind to your patients, your colleagues and yourself.

Case study – GP Principal, Clinical Director and Chief Medical Officer

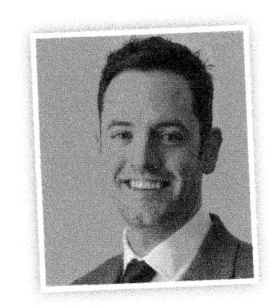

Dr Dan Bunstone MBChB MRCGP MAE
GP Principal, Chapelford Medical Centre, Warrington
Clinical Director, Warrington Innovation Network
Chief Medical Officer, Push Doctor and Speed Medical Examination Services
Previously Chair of Warrington CCG

What attracted you to general practice?

I was initially attracted to a career as a GP by the opportunity it afforded me to have a truly portfolio career. I love the freedom to work on different areas and have a genuinely varied week.

Having the opportunity to make a difference to large systems and influence the strategic direction for organisations is a real privilege and one that I do not take lightly. The real appeal for me is that I always find myself thinking and strategizing: how to do things better, looking for gaps and opportunities, and ways of enabling collaboration between different organisations. That is massive for me and a real energy generator. Around 2 years after qualifying as a GP, I was appointed as a CCG Board member for Warrington CCG, and 4 years later I was appointed as Chair. I began to do medicolegal work and was appointed as clinical lead for Speed Medical before being appointed as the Chief Medical Officer. After that, came the opportunity to work as the Chief Medical Officer of Push Doctor.

What are the drawbacks of general practice?

I suppose one of the drawbacks is that there is always something seeming to be happening. As a rule of thumb, two half-time roles will always add up to more than one full-time role. I enjoy that aspect of things, but it isn't for everybody. Managing all of the commitments and making everything fit can be a challenge, but this is something you get used to, and soon it becomes second nature. If it doesn't, then it might mean it's not for you. Nevertheless, I find that any potential drawbacks are far outweighed by the benefits.

What is your advice for those considering general practice?

Try everything, and don't ever close your mind to opportunity. If you try something and it's not for you, then move onto the next thing. You'll never regret the skill set you have gained through the journey, and it will very likely be useful again in the future in one guise or other. The caveat is though, you don't keep trying everything forever. Find the things you are good at, which give you energy and purpose, and if you find that nectar of a role that you would work in even if you weren't being paid, then you've made it!

CHAPTER 16

Alternative careers

So much can be accomplished by working as a doctor in the NHS. All UK medical school graduates should recognise this and be appreciative of the opportunities they have. For the majority of medical school graduates, working within the NHS will allow them to achieve their career goals. However, this is not representative of everyone. In this chapter we will discuss some of the career paths that deviate from the conventional method of training. We have chosen our top five for you, but remember, there are many more careers out there you may wish to explore.

16.1 Military doctor

It is possible to work as a doctor in the UK armed forces. Substantial financial support is available for medical students who sign up to the Army, Navy or Air Force. In return, they must serve a minimum period in the armed forces. Those who fail to carry out their commitments may be required to return their financial support. The general advantages of working in the armed forces are that it allows you to travel with work, offers better pay (especially when taking medical student bursaries and subsidised living costs into account), exposure to armed forces work and machinery (including combat training and weaponry), guaranteed leadership training, a lot of exercise, and it allows you to socialise regularly with interesting people. Time spent as a doctor in the armed forces can also set you up nicely for a career in the following specialties: general practice, emergency medicine, anaesthetics and resuscitation, general surgery, general medicine, psychiatry, pathology, radiology, rheumatology and rehabilitation, occupational medicine and public health. The general drawbacks of working in the armed forces are that it is not well suited to careers in specialties that have not been listed above, it is a big commitment, time must be spent away from family and friends, restricted freedom of location, and potentially hazardous work if deployed. If you are interested in working as a doctor in the armed forces, please read some of the highlights for each of the armed forces below:

16.1.1 Army

- **Entry points:** during medical school/after FY2/when a qualified GP or consultant.

- **Medical student bursaries:** £10,000 per year for the last 3 years of study.

- **Additional financial support:** £45,000 grant after completing the Professionally Qualified Officer (PQO) course at Sandhurst.

- **Commitment period:** Short Service Commission is for 8 years. However, it is possible to opt out at the initial commitment point at 4 years after commencement of officer training.

- **Medical student eligibility:** to sign-up you must be a British, Commonwealth, or Irish citizen who studies at a UK university, and is within 3 years of graduation.

- **Website:** https://apply.army.mod.uk/roles/army-medical-service/doctor.

16.1.2 Royal Navy

- **Medical student bursaries:** a salary of £16,797 is provided for the final 3 years of medical school, plus full payment of tuition fees, and a book allowance.

- **Selection process:** interview and performance testing.

- **Training:** 7 weeks must be spent at a Royal Naval College.

- **Commitment period:** Short Service Commission is for 6 years from completion of FY1.

- **Website:** www.royalnavy.mod.uk/careers/roles-and-specialisations/services/surface-fleet/medical-officer-cadet.

16.1.3 Royal Air Force

- **Medical student bursaries:** £3000 a year for years 2 and 3 of studies, plus a salary of £14,983 – £16,823 and tuition fees

ALTERNATIVE CAREERS

payment for the final 2 years of study. A book allowance is also accessible.

- **Training:** you must become a member of the University Air Squadron, where you will receive free flying lessons.
- **Commitment period:** 6 or 12 years from completion of FY1.
- **Website:** ✔ www.raf.mod.uk/recruitment/roles/roles-finder/medical-and-medical-support/medical-officer.

Case study – RAF doctor

| Flt Lt Dr Charles Badu-Boateng MBBS BSc (Hons) |
| Medical Officer, RAF |
| Internal Medicine Trainee (IMT2) |

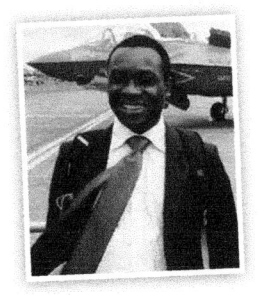

What attracted you to your chosen career path?

The opportunity to go beyond the standard medical career and to deliver high quality care under demanding but rewarding conditions. There is a strong emphasis on personal development and the fostering of excellent leadership and military skills that remain transferable to everyday life. We are offered opportunities and encouragement to engage in adventure training, as well as supported to compete in high level professional sports. A great chance to travel the world (and around the UK) whilst in service. Brilliant lifelong friends.

What are the drawbacks of your chosen career path?

Typically it will take a little longer to become a consultant or a GP in comparison to civilian colleagues. It can be challenging to meet clinical training requirements on top of military duties. From FY1 to ST2 years, location for training is fairly limited and may not fit into personal and family plans (this gets better with higher specialty training).

What is your advice for those considering becoming a military doctor?

Medicine is a truly rewarding career in so many different ways. However, military medicine takes it up a notch. Resilience is an important quality to foster; it may not come naturally but can certainly be developed. Ensure you speak to current trainees and Defence Consultant Advisors for the specialty you are interested in to get an idea of what to expect. Physical fitness is important. Just do it; military medicine is far more flexible than it used to be, and family friendly too!

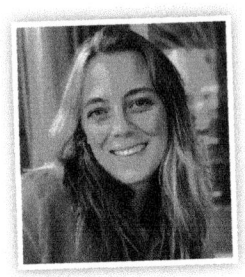

Case study – Army doctor

Dr Rhiannon Austin MBChB BSc
Army doctor, FY2

What attracted you to your chosen career path?

Being able to incorporate hobbies that I love into working life; the military promotes an active and outdoor-based lifestyle. As part of your job, you are encouraged to keep fit and develop new skills constantly and there are always courses and opportunities for 'adventurous training' available (though not usually during FY1 and FY2). There is a strong focus on non-clinical as well as clinical skills, for example, leadership and communication skills are constantly being developed. A lot of people talk about a sense of belonging in the military, you live in the mess with the other foundation doctors, spend a lot of time together and as a result often become a close-knit group. The military also provides a real sense of comradeship and people will often go out of their way to help you.

What are the drawbacks of your chosen career path?

Commitment to a certain number of years once you sign up to the army, so you have to be sure at that point that it's what you want to do for those next few years. There are also a limited number of hospitals to choose from for FY1 and FY2 and a limited number of specialty training pathways to choose from. You can do general practice, A&E, anaesthetics, core medical or core surgical training; however most other training pathways are not offered by the military. Whilst a career in the military does offer lots of exciting opportunities, you have little flexibility and bargaining power over things such as where you get placed and when you get deployed or posted. You have to be prepared to be completely flexible with your plans in this sense.

What is your advice for those considering becoming a military doctor?

The military is a lifestyle, not just a career path. As such, it is not for everyone. Try to talk to people in the military to see if it appeals to you. The application process to get into the military is a lengthy process (approximately 1 year), involving lots of different stages, so if you are seriously considering it then it is a good idea to get the initial paperwork in sooner rather than later. You get a bit of a flavour of the military through the various stages so you can get an idea of whether the military is for you through the application process itself. Don't take a decision to join the military lightly, if you find it is not for you further down the line then it is difficult to get out of it.

Case study – Navy doctor

Anonymous Navy doctor, MBBS, MSc, BSc (hons)
Surgeon Lieutenant

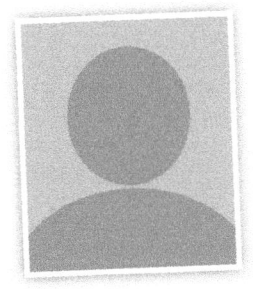

What attracted you to your chosen career path?

As a military doctor, once you complete your two foundation years in hospital, you go away to Officer training. After this, you serve a period of two and a half years (or half a year in the RAF) as a GDMO (general duties medical officer), in which you act as the doctor for your unit, whether it be on land or sea, at home or on foreign soil. The attraction of this, for me, was the opportunity to travel to interesting places around the world, test myself physically and psychologically, be exposed to difficult medical scenarios, make lifelong friends and learn new skills outside of the medical umbrella. After this GDMO period you return to the UK and begin your specialty training. Once this is complete, depending on the specialty you have chosen, you will again get the opportunity to practise medicine/surgery/anaesthetics/primary care, etc. away from your UK-based place of work. This then gives you the opportunity to hone your skills in your particular field but in more extreme and challenging environments.

What are the drawbacks of your chosen career path?

Due to the GDMO period, you are held back from starting your specialty training for 1 or 3 years (depending on the service you join) compared to your civilian colleagues who begin after FY2 if they do not take an FY3 year. I perceive this as a good opportunity to enjoy practising medicine in the military, whereas those who want to expedite their career might be put off by this. Naturally, you need to consider the dangerous and potentially life-threatening aspects of the job, as well as the time spent away from family and loved ones.

What is your advice for those considering becoming a military doctor?

Try to get in contact with a current military trainee, as we are generally the best people to ask about the ins and outs of the job. I have close friends from across all three services, as most of us do, so we can give you a fairly good picture of what to expect across each service.

16.2 Entrepreneurship

It is becoming increasingly popular for doctors to create a start-up business as a source of additional income. This usually begins as a spare-time endeavour and is managed whilst working as a full-time doctor. However, as the business grows, some choose to become part-time doctors or leave the profession altogether. There are many advantages to being a doctor when entering the business world. Doctors are widely regarded as intelligent, determined and trustworthy people who work well in teams. They also often have valuable insight from working in the healthcare industry. If you are interested in entrepreneurship opportunities specifically for doctors, including internships or full-time roles with start-up businesses or accelerator funding for your own start-up have a look at ✔ **www.opportunities.doctorpreneurs.com**. Recent trends in entrepreneurial activity amongst doctors include creating apps, performing cosmetic procedures and building social media accounts. Notable examples include ✔ **www.geekymedics.com**, ✔ **www.dr-toolbox.com**, ✔ **www.mdcalc.com**, ✔ **www.hellopando.com**, @drpimplepopper, @laradevganmd, @thefoodmedic, @doctors_kitchen, @drfrankiejs.

Many doctors seek out formal training to help with becoming a successful entrepreneur, for example:
- the NHS England Clinical Entrepreneur Training Programme
- undertaking a Master of Business Administration (MBA).

16.2.1 NHS England clinical entrepreneur training programme

This is open to health professionals who wish to develop an entrepreneurial venture alongside their clinical commitments. The programme provides support for its participants in many ways, including: mentoring and coaching, placements and internships, facilitation of relationships with commercial organisations, educational events, funding signposting and networking events. Entry to the programme is competitive and decided by CV quality and interview performance.

16.2.2 Master of Business Administration

An MBA is typically open to those with a 2:1 undergraduate degree (or higher) and a minimum of 3 years of managerial experience. It is designed to prepare individuals for life as a manager or CEO. Modules are usually based on themes such as leadership and management, economics, finance, business strategy, marketing, supply chain management, innovation, international business, entrepreneurship, and brand management. The full-time degree takes a year to complete. However, there are also options to complete part-time MBA programmes (over 2 years) and online MBA programmes (in your spare time). MBA programmes conclude with a dissertation or work-based project, which requires you to draw upon all of the knowledge you have gained through the curriculum. Many MBA students use this as an opportunity to create a written business model for their intended start-up.

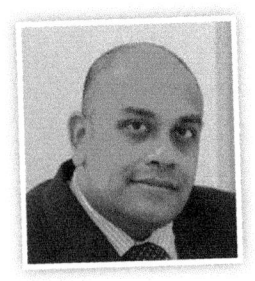

Case study – Founder and CEO

Johann Malawana
Founder and CEO, Medics.Academy
Founder and Managing Director, The Healthcare Leadership Academy
Education & Training Lead, Healthcare UK – Department for International Trade
Honorary Senior Clinical Lecturer, UCLan Medical School
Former Obstetrician in the NHS

What attracted you to entrepreneurship?

I want to make the world a better place. That might sound a bit simplistic or obvious, but I believe I can make a bigger impact on the world and improve the lives of more people by solving the challenges and problems I am working on, than any other option I personally have. I enjoy my work to the point I often don't think of it as work. I like solving problems and I like guiding and mentoring people. Most of all, I get to surround myself with an incredibly talented group of people that inspire me every day to make a concerted effort to change the world around me. I get to help some of the best early-stage healthcare clinicians to find their path in the world and that is incredibly invigorating and empowering.

What are the drawbacks of entrepreneurship?

A lot of hard work and long hours. When you run your own organisation or when you are doing academic work, there is less job security. Ultimately, you are responsible for people's jobs, so you can never really take time off. When I used to finish a day of work as an obstetrician, there would be residual concerns for my patients, but generally when you left the hospital, you could turn your focus elsewhere. It isn't really the same in many of my current roles.

ALTERNATIVE CAREERS   CHAPTER 16

What is your advice for those considering entrepreneurship?

If you want to innovate, get on with it. Stop waiting for someone to give you permission. Surround yourself with talented people and find the most inspiring people you can to work with. If you are looking for an alternative career because you don't like medicine, be aware that the grass is not always greener on the other side of the fence. Medicine is the absolute best career you can have. It is rewarding, you gain incredible amounts of social credibility and respect and it is relatively well paid. You should explore alternatives as a positive choice rather than as a negative. If you have a negative reason, solve whatever the root cause of that is, as you may find the switch may not give you what you want.

Case study – Junior doctor and CEO

Dr Michael Watts MBChB BSc (Hons)
Junior Doctor in the NHS
CEO of a health software development company: Blüm Health Ltd
Current MBA student
NHS Clinical Entrepreneurship Fellow
Medical Director Fellowship in Digital Communication

What attracted you to entrepreneurship?

Throughout my time at medical school, I realised that there was an opportunity to help people on a larger scale, rather than patient-by-patient. With my particular interest in technology, it felt natural to harness my two passions as one. Through this, I am now able to turn innovative ideas into impactful technology that will touch the lives of patients throughout the nation and beyond. I continue to work as a doctor and plan to do so for as long as I can.

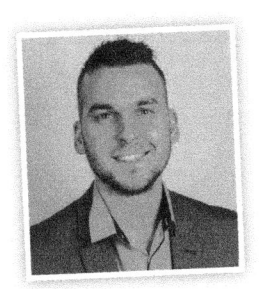

What are the drawbacks of entrepreneurship?

Some will see this as a drawback, but I see this as also exciting, but the task of developing something that is completely new and innovative carries risks. Fortunately, as a clinician you have a good amount of job security which enables some risk mitigation. Nevertheless, taking that leap of faith is difficult. Once you do, you then have the complexity of managing both clinical and non-clinical duties, but this is something that we (as clinicians) learn to do well during the early years of our career.

What is your advice for those considering entrepreneurship?

John Rockefeller said, "don't be afraid to give up the good to go for the great". Better still, don't give up the good either. I am striking a balance of maintaining my good (I love being a doctor) but my great is large scale change to the NHS. Many people around you will question what you are doing, why you would put yourself through it, but ultimately "you can't climb the ladder of success with your hands in your pockets" (Arnold Schwarzenegger). Decide what success looks like for you, whether that be becoming a consultant, being able to travel the world, or impact the lives of millions. More important still, ensure you enjoy it, surround yourself with like-minded people, and keep a healthy work–life balance at all times.

16.3 Pharmaceutical physician

There is a recognised pathway for doctors who wish to become pharmaceutical physicians. The majority of doctors who make the transition from NHS to pharmaceutical companies will work in medical affairs. This means they are tasked with turning scientific information into sustainable clinical practice. There are also opportunities for pharmaceutical physicians to become involved in research, development of new medicines, marketing of medicines, and work at regulatory authorities. Working within the pharmaceutical industry provides an opportunity for doctors to climb the corporate ladder, work for international companies and achieve good job satisfaction.

To begin this journey, doctors can search for pharmaceutical physician jobs by reading the careers section of medical journals such as *BMJ Careers*. Furthermore, there are specialist pharmaceutical recruitment firms that can be approached, for example, **www.agencycentral.co.uk/agencysearch/pharm/agencysearch.htm**. Networking with industry professionals and utilising LinkedIn are also recommended ways of gaining information about pharmaceutical physician roles. Whilst working in the industry, it is beneficial for pharmaceutical physicians to undertake formal education and training in pharmaceutical medicine. Those who complete the pharmaceutical medicine specialty training (PMST) programme are able to become a pharmaceutical medicine consultant. The PMST is a four-year competency-based programme that is centred in the workplace. The curriculum includes the Diploma in Pharmaceutical Medicine and the specialty knowledge that is required to progress in the industry. The eligibility criteria for doctors undertaking the PMST are as follows:

- Holds a valid GMC registration with a licence to practise
- Is employed by a UK-based pharmaceutical organisation that is a GMC-approved PMST location
- Has a minimum of 4 years of clinical experience
- Has a GMC-approved Educational Supervisor in pharmaceutical medicine
- Meets the person specifications for pharmaceutical ST3 entry on the HEE website: **https://specialtytraining.hee.nhs.uk/Recruitment/Person-specifications**.

Doctors who decide to work for a pharmaceutical company can expect a salary that is at least equal to their NHS wage. In addition to this, they may receive annual benefits such as a performance-based bonus, private health insurance, and a company car. Further information can be found at:

- www.bmj.com/content/347/bmj.f6977
- www.bma.org.uk/media/1772/bma-pharmaceutical-physican-sept-2013.pdf
- www.abpi.org.uk/media/4554/pharmaceutical_careers_for_doctors_in_the_uk_october_2017.pdf.

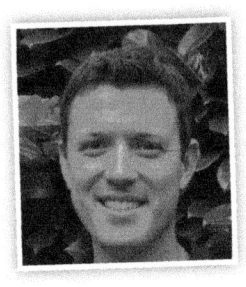

Case study – Senior medical advisor

Dr Peter Morgan-Warren BMBCh MA (Oxon) PhD FRCOphth
Senior Medical Advisor (ophthalmology), Bayer PLC
Former Royal Air Force Medical Officer, Specialty Registrar in Ophthalmology, and Medical Assessor at the MHRA

What attracted you to pharmaceutical medicine?

My career path decisions have been shaped by interest, opportunity and circumstances at particular stages of my career so far. I was drawn to ophthalmology by an interest in visual sciences, an analytical eye for detail, and engaging with a medical specialty incorporating elements of medicine and surgery, acute and chronic conditions, and all age groups. More recently, a developing interest and opportunity to apply my experience in the regulatory and pharmaceutical sector has influenced my career direction away from clinical practice.

What are the drawbacks of pharmaceutical medicine?

It certainly has not been predetermined, and I have had a few changes of direction along the way. This is not an approach that would fit comfortably for everyone. Each major move, e.g. clinical practice into research (PhD), clinical work into the regulatory sector and then into the pharmaceutical industry, has involved a steep learning curve and the requirement for development and application of new skills and approaches.

What is your advice for those considering pharmaceutical medicine?

Don't consider my career path – consider your own! I would certainly recommend choosing a direction you are comfortable with, and remember that it is never too late to change direction if things don't work out as hoped or planned. Understand and recognise your own interests, skills, circumstances and areas to develop, and don't be afraid to seek honest advice (from as many people who are prepared to give it) to help influence your own choices.

Case study – Consultant pharmaceutical physician

Dr Mayur R Joshi MBBS, BSc, DPM, AICSM, MFPM
Consultant Pharmaceutical Physician
Global Medical Head, Retina – Novartis
Editor, *Journal of the Faculty of Pharmaceutical Medicine*

What attracted you to pharmaceutical medicine?

After working in the NHS, I realised I wanted to learn more about healthcare systems and how I can influence them better. As a doctor working in the NHS, you are able to have an impact on your patients, but it is difficult to have a more widespread impact. This led me to research alternative career options. I was proud to be a medic and wanted to retain the relevance of my training and qualifications. In the end, pharmaceutical medicine was very interesting to me, particularly, rare diseases, advanced therapies, and bringing novel medicines to market. These areas provide an opportunity to help people who have not been able to receive help previously. I wanted to work in a commercial environment as I was business-minded and wanted to experiment at work. Clinical research and health economics outcomes research were also attractive aspects. Lastly, I realised working in pharmaceutical medicine would provide me with an opportunity for less rigid career progression.

What are the drawbacks of pharmaceutical medicine?

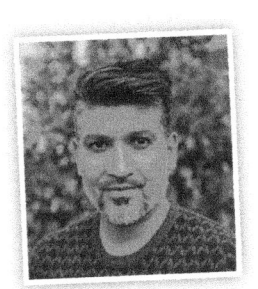

When working within a corporate environment you must align with the company's strategies. Some roles are product focused. These roles may not be as attractive as others and can prevent you from exploring other aspects of the business. Medical teams are not typically incentivised by revenue. However, revenue is crucial for the company. There is also a lot of necessary admin and compliance with regulations which can be restrictive and tiresome.

What is your advice for those considering pharmaceutical medicine?

Regardless of the industry you want to move into, think deep down about what your motivations are. Are you running away from the NHS? Or is there a genuine attraction to the industry you are going into? It's okay to be uninspired by the NHS. However, don't let this be your reason for leaving medicine without understanding your next industry and discovering it is something that inspires you. Prepare to be the novice in your new industry and maintain a curious mindset.

16.4 Management consulting

If you have a natural interest in business and want to step away from clinical practice, then perhaps management consulting is the career for you. The role of a management consultant is to solve business-hindering problems for organisations. This is done by providing expert business advice and equipping organisations to maintain a high level of operating performance. Doctors who make the switch will usually begin in an analyst role. Analysts are mostly responsible for collecting and analysing data. With time and hard work, analysts are promoted to consultant roles. The next step up is to senior consultant or managerial roles. At this stage, work will involve designing projects and ensuring they are completed successfully by leading teams.

Management consulting firms provide services for companies across a wide range of industries and sectors. Examples include non-profit organisations, the public sector and government, financial services, manufacturing, hospitality and leisure, media, retail and healthcare. As a doctor entering the industry, you are able to specialise in any of these areas. Most doctors will decide to utilise their medical knowledge and specialise in healthcare, which involves providing expert advice to the NHS, private hospitals, pharmaceutical companies and medical device organisations. Business-minded doctors are often attracted to management consulting by the potential salary and work–life balance. To begin with, salaries are similar to those earned in the NHS, but they have the potential to quickly exceed NHS salaries. Further, management consultants tend to work long days from Monday to Friday but do not work night shifts, weekends, Christmas, New Year or bank holidays.

The journey can begin by searching for vacancies online. There are many jobsites that advertise for management consulting analyst roles, for example: ➤ **www.consultancy.uk/jobs** and ➤ **www.glassdoor.co.uk/index.htm**. Furthermore, it is always useful to visit management consulting company websites to see what recruitment opportunities are available. The big names in the industry are Accenture, Boston Consulting Group, Deloitte, Ernst & Young, KPMG, McKinsey, PA Consulting, and PwC. LinkedIn is also a useful resource for discovering recruitment opportunities. Candidates will be expected to provide a high-quality CV. Generally, management consulting firms are looking for candidates who have a history of academic success, an evidenced interest in business, leadership skills, and a proven ability to analyse data. A portion of candidates will then be selected for interview. Each firm handles this process differently. However, it is common practice to test each candidate's analytical and problem-solving abilities during interview. This usually involves use of a case study and a series of related questions. It is crucial to prepare for this part of the interview and there are many helpful resources available online and in bookshops, for example, ➤ **www.myconsultingcoach.com/case-interview** and ➤ **www.igotanoffer.com/blogs/mckinsey-case-interview-blog/case-interview**.

If you would like to sample the working life of a management consultant before leaping away from medicine, PwC provides a taster week for doctors and final year medical students. This allows clinicians to work within the M&A strategy team on projects related to healthcare, pharmaceuticals and life sciences. Business concepts training is also provided to enhance the level of insight gained.

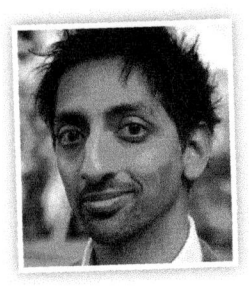

Case study – Medical director

Dr Tapas Mukherjee MBChB MRCP DipMedEd
Medical Director at Havas Lynx Europe
Former respiratory registrar and education fellow
NHS clinical staff member for 13 years

What attracted you to your chosen career path?

The grass always seems greener on the other side of the fence. You always feel like you're being hard done by, no matter what job you're in. Despite feeling very capable and having a lot of autonomy in the NHS, there is a narrow selection of fields to choose from and there are limitations to what you can do. Those who have interests that are not aligned with the traditional interest of NHS trainees might find it unclear where to focus a lot of their energy. Luckily, I was offered the opportunity to combine my medical knowledge and experience with my interests in an exciting and secure way. The reason I decided against maintaining a part-time clinical role was to ensure my full commitment and to avoid the stigma attached to part-time work.

What are the drawbacks of your chosen career path?

You have to be very senior or sought after to achieve a high salary outside of the NHS. You are also not guaranteed a pension that matches your NHS one. I work just as hard in my new role as I did in the NHS. I also work similar hours due to travel; business trips mean you spend less time with your family. Even though I now get looked after much better by my company, there will always be work-related stress. If you don't perform or keep reinventing yourself, you risk being fired as there is always someone who can replace you. In the NHS there is a lot of job security and you will always have a job for life.

What is your advice for those considering management consulting?

Be mindful that 'working in the NHS' is a world-class and world-recognised badge. Losing the badge is not the end of the world because there are other credible jobs. However, the NHS badge is unique and when someone says they have worked in the NHS for a number of years, they have a very credible voice. If you're very early in your career and considering jumping ship, people can see through this. You risk becoming a young person with a good degree who has dabbled in a bit of medicine. If you completely leave the NHS it is difficult to return. Make sure you're leaving for the right reasons and that you understand what you're giving up. If you're not sure, there is no harm staying in the NHS for a bit longer because these job opportunities will still be there.

16.5 Medico-legal careers

There are roles for doctors who wish to become involved in medical law. Eligibility for each role mostly depends on how much clinical experience you have as a doctor. If this amounts to less than 5 years, there may be roles within NHS Trusts such as inquests and claims handler. This is not a recognised training path for doctors. Therefore, combination with less-than-full-time clinical training is not usually an option and maintaining GMC registration becomes your responsibility.

If you have more than 5 years of clinical experience, there are medico-legal adviser roles within medical defence organisations (e.g. Medical Defence Union and Medical Protection Society) that you may wish to consider. Candidates are expected to have achieved a postgraduate legal qualification (e.g. Medical Law LLM) or gained experience in medico-legal work. These roles can be full-time or can be combined with less-than-full-time clinical training. GMC registration is a medico-legal adviser job requirement and so your employing defence organisation will assist with maintaining your registration.

If your clinical experience amounts to more than 10 years, there are expert witness roles that might interest you. This involves using your knowledge and experience as a clinician to provide an independent opinion on clinical negligence claims. You must submit this opinion to a solicitor by writing a report which takes into account all of the clinical documentation and relevant publications that are available. Following this, you may be required to attend the trial and take into account other evidence before providing a statement.

A career in medical law is able to provide doctors with variety from standard clinical practice. It is a career that appeals to doctors with strong literacy skills and a desire for justice. These are just a few examples of roles within medical law and if you are interested in investigating this career path further, visit ✔ **www.medicfootprints.org/a-guide-to-a-medico-legal-career-for-doctors/**. You should also utilise your network and LinkedIn to find a mentor who has experience in this field.

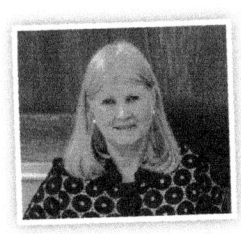

Case study – Expert witness

Dr Frances Cranfield MBBS LLM LRCP MRCS DRCOG DFSRH DFMS DMJ RCPathME FFFLM FRCGP
General Practitioner – Senior partner
Member of RCGP Council
Observer on BMA General Practitioners Committee
Founder Member of the Expert Witness Institute and the Faculty of Forensic & Legal Medicine of the Royal College of Physicians
Former President of the Clinical Forensic & Legal Medicine Section of the Royal Society of Medicine
Assistant Coroner Hertfordshire

What attracted you to medical law?

Chance initially. My practice acted as forensic medical examiners and I was then invited to join a committee of one of the major medical protection organisations. I became an expert witness, including for the Shipman Inquiry and the first case of gross medical negligence against a GP, and was subsequently appointed assistant coroner. I love the mix of work and the ability to bring skills and knowledge from one field of work to another and the chance to make a difference in so many different areas. Expert witness work is stimulating, educational and challenging and has some flexibility.

What are the drawbacks of medical law?

The downside is that the workload can be unpredictable and that as an expert witness or indeed a forensic medical examiner you can be open to challenge and criticisms in open court. Another downside of expert witness work is the court trial windows which can make planning in life difficult. As a coroner or medical examiner, you are frequently dealing with the darkest and most distressing times of people's lives and whilst it is a great privilege, self-care is also vital.

What is your advice for those considering medical law?

Life is full of opportunities and it is a case of picking the right one for you. If you want to do it, have the courage to take that first step. Find support (a mentor) and make time and space. The variety of a portfolio medico-legal career can reduce the risk of burnout. There are many medico-legal opportunities including forensic medical examiners, expert witnesses, medico-legal advisors, and although it is no longer possible to become a coroner unless a practising lawyer, there will soon to be the opportunity to be a medical examiner, to deal with deaths not reported to the coroner.

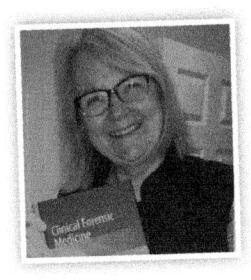

Case study – Forensic medical examiner

Dr Margaret M Stark LLM MSc(Med Ed) MB BS FFFLM FACBS FHEA FACLM FRCP FFCFM (RCPA) RCPathME DGM DMJ DAB

President, Faculty of Forensic & Legal Medicine of the Royal College of Physicians (FFLM). Forensic Physician (Forensic Medical Examiner Metropolitan Police Service and expert witness). Appraiser.

Responsible Officer Care & Custody (Health) Ltd. Deputy Medical Referee, Croydon Crematorium. Chairman Forensic Science & Training & Education Sub-Committees (FFLM). Lead Facilitator Training Course in GFM (FFLM & University of Teesside). Educational Advisor (FFLM examinations).

Former Principal in General Practice.

What attracted you to medical law?

The unpredictability of working with the police. No two days are the same. I have been involved in some amazing cases in London and worked for 3 years as Head of the Clinical Forensic Medicine Unit for New South Wales Police Force based in Sydney. I also love the interaction with the law and the medico-legal and ethical problems that arise from the clinical work. I am self-employed so in charge of my own destiny, but that has its drawbacks (see below). Overall, I prefer being my own boss. The law degree helped me write prose properly again and it really helps having been trained to read (and understand) legal documents. I enjoy the 'theatre' of court work. I love to teach/train and doing a formal course in medical education was so much fun. I enjoy all the roles outlined above and they all seem to dovetail into each other. Also, I relished the challenge of setting up a new Faculty covering clinical forensic medicine in the UK and Australasia.

What are the drawbacks of medical law?

Lack of specialty status for forensic and legal medicine. Lack of recognition for what we do. Working as a sole trader in the independent/private sector I have no holiday pay, sick pay or pension; it is easier to be employed with a regular salary and allowances, whereas if I don't work, I don't get paid. Underestimation of the amount of charity work required in setting up the FFLM!

What is your advice for those considering medical law?

Aim for a portfolio career so that if one aspect doesn't work out you have training and experience in another area of practice, e.g. general practice or emergency medicine in combination with forensic and legal medicine. Consider ideas outside mainstream medicine that can enhance your career such as a formal teaching qualification, experience and qualifications in business administration, photography, life coaching, etc.

Case study – Assistant coroner

Mr Leslie Hamilton LLM FRCSEng FRCSEd(C-Th).
Assistant Coroner in Durham
Retired Consultant Cardiac Surgeon in Newcastle

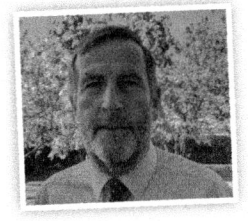

What attracted you to your chosen career path?

Paediatric/congenital heart surgery brought all my early interests together. I found the interaction with parents very rewarding. Giving evidence to the Bristol Inquiry (Google it) stimulated my interest in the legal aspects of practice and prompted me to undertake an LLM in Medical Law during my time as a Consultant. This gave me an opportunity to teach on a legal course at the Royal College of Surgeons and opened the doors to the world of Coroners... and a subsequent appointment as Assistant Coroner.

What are the drawbacks of your chosen career path?

Paediatric cardiac surgery is undertaken in too many units in the country (see ◂ **www.rcseng.ac.uk/news-and-events/blog/heart-surgery-reconfiguration**) and so there are only 2 or 3 surgeons in each unit. This means a heavy physical, mental and emotional burden on each surgeon. I was able to stop and continue as an adult cardiac surgeon (I had a mixed post because I had trained in both) but this is no longer possible. Appointments now are full time paediatric cardiac surgery. I do not know how the current generation of paediatric cardiac surgeons will cope as they 'mature' into their late 50s and 60s.

What is your advice for those considering a career in surgery or medical law?

Do what you really enjoy but have plans to have a different direction later – medical practice will change dramatically over the time of your career. Be on the lookout for opening doors.

16.6 Top tips for medical students

- If a career in the armed forces is right for you, **do not miss out on the financial support** that is available to medical students.

- If you create a start-up company, **seek expert help**. For example, if you have an idea for a medical mobile app, team up with a software expert. Many entrepreneurs make the mistake of trying to do everything themselves.

- **Intercalation may be a great opportunity** to complete a degree that will boost your career prospects in one of these alternative fields.

- **Reach out to doctors with experience in your desired career.** They are the best people to ask for advice regarding benefits/drawbacks of the job, tips for how to prepare your CV and secure a job. They may also be able to signpost you to other careers that might be better suited to you.

- For more information on alternative careers including civil service, expedition medicine, medical journalism, politics and healthcare in prisons, see ➤ **www.healthcareers.nhs.uk/explore-roles/doctors/career-opportunities-doctors/alternative-roles-doctors**.

CHAPTER 17

Working abroad

One of the great perks to a career in medicine is having the opportunity to work abroad. During medical school, you will be given the chance to experience this as part of your medical elective. After graduating, you may wish to experience this again. Opportunities abroad exist in many forms. There are voluntary roles for doctors within non-profit organisations such as Médecins Sans Frontières, Raleigh International, Africa Health Placements, and Blue Ventures. These organisations all provide clear recruitment information on their websites. In addition to these roles, there are paid roles for doctors within foreign health services, which can be on either a temporary or permanent basis. The relevant recruitment information for these roles can be difficult to find online. In this chapter, we will cover the most valuable points for doctors who are considering working in the USA, Canada, Australia, and New Zealand. We will also discuss the most important considerations for doctors planning to return to work in the UK. Foreign travel is currently subject to government-enforced COVID-19 travel restrictions, so please remember to check official government websites for the most accurate and up-to-date advice:
- www.gov.uk/guidance/travel-advice-novel-coronavirus and
- www.gov.uk/foreign-travel-advice.

17.1 The USA

The first step for doctors who wish to practise in the USA is to gain certification from the Educational Commission for Foreign Medical Graduates (ECFMG). Providing that you have graduated or will soon graduate from an approved medical school, you must pass the following examinations:
- United States Medical Licensing Examination (USMLE) Step 1 (basic medical)
- USMLE Step 2 (clinical knowledge)
- USMLE Step 2 (clinical skills).

The first two examinations listed can be completed before graduating medical school. All three must be completed within a 7-year period to receive an ECFMG certificate. Once this has been achieved, you can then secure an employment visa (either temporary or settlement) and are eligible to enter a Graduate Medical Education (GME) programme, also known as a residency programme. These programmes are comparable to higher specialty training in the UK. Residencies last between 3 and 7 years, depending on the specialty. It may be possible to have the residency duration reduced if you have already completed some overseas specialist training. The American Medical Association recommends that overseas doctors enrol in observership placements prior to applying to residencies. This allows overseas doctors to gain a solid understanding of the work that will be involved. After completing the first year of a residency, most doctors will look to complete USMLE Part 3. Passing this exam enables doctors to gain a licence to practise once they have completed their residency. The purpose of USMLE Part 3 is to assess if a doctor is able to safely practise medicine in an unsupervised environment. If a specialist consultant in the UK wishes to practise in the USA, it may be possible for them to liaise with the relevant US specialty board and bypass some of the residency programme. Specialty boards are comparable to Royal Colleges in the UK. To become certified by a specialty board, doctors are required to pass examinations; this is a voluntary process but may be required for certain roles.

17.2 Canada

The process of becoming a registered doctor in Canada varies depending on the province or territory, and so doctors should contact the medical regulatory authority of the province or territory in which they want to work. This approach will help provide accurate and relevant information about international medical graduate (IMG) entry requirements.

To demonstrate the standard of knowledge required to practise medicine in Canada, applicants must pass the Medical Council of Canada Qualifying Examination (MCCQE). Applicants are then expected to provide their medical credential documents to the Medical Council of Canada's Physician Credentials Repository (PCRC). Once the documents have been accepted and approved, they will be held indefinitely by the repository and can be used for future job applications. Doctors must then complete an accredited postgraduate training programme, also known as residency training. This will last 2 years for Family Medicine and 4–5 years for other specialties. Entry to these programmes is usually via the Canadian Resident Matching Service (CaRMS) or IMG-specific programmes. Applications to IMG-specific programmes are assessed with regard to examinations, portfolios and interviews. Successful applicants can request a work permit from the Canadian High Commission.

Throughout residency training, doctors practise under an educational licence and are not permitted to work independently. Doctors must pass the MCCQE Parts I and II to practise independently. This is irrespective of the doctor's specialty. Part II can only be taken after completing a minimum of 12 months of residency training. Upon completion of a residency training programme, doctors are eligible to sit the certification examination specific to their specialty. It may be possible for doctors who have already completed specialist training in the UK to bypass residency training and sit the relevant certification examinations straight away. Afterwards, all that might remain to gain a licence to practise medicine in Canada is fulfilment of a return-of-service agreement. This involves practising in an underserviced area for a set amount of time.

17.3 Australia

The UK medical school training system is considered equivalent to the one in Australia. Therefore, UK medical school graduates do not have to sit additional examinations to practise medicine in Australia. To gain limited registration from the Australian Health Practitioner Regulation Agency (AHPRA), UK medical school graduates must have a licence to practise in the UK (gained after completing FY1) and must be of good standing with the GMC and their employers. They must also have a job offer in Australia and have completed the Australian Medical Council (AMC) registration process via the 'Competent Authority Pathway'. Limited registration with the AHPRA allows UK doctors to work under the supervision of a senior medical practitioner. Usually, after a period of 12 months, if the supervisor raises no concerns, UK doctors can apply for full registration. Note that limited registration with the AHPRA is given for a specific job, and so UK doctors must reapply if changing jobs. If a doctor has already completed some specialist training in the UK, they should liaise with the relevant Australian Specialist Medical College and Medical Board to gain limited registration to work in their specialty.

There are many ways to find jobs in Australia. Roles can be found in journals such as the *BMJ* and the *Medical Journal of Australia*. They can also be sourced through medical recruitment firms and locum agencies. If you wish to take a more direct approach, states in Australia advertise jobs for doctors via centralised application websites, such as ➤ **www.health.nsw.gov.au/jmo/Pages/default.aspx**. This requires a regular effort to browse through vacancies and identify which ones are relevant. Another direct approach is to contact the medical workforce department in hospitals of interest to you and provide them with a CV. If you opt for this method, remember that persistence is key. In Australia, the training year for junior doctors commences in February. Jobs beginning in February are advertised around July and offers are usually made by October. There are also jobs that start 6 months after the typical start date in February. These jobs are generally preferable for UK doctors, because an August start date coincides with the UK training year. If you are applying for jobs that begin in August, it is advisable to start applying around November. This leaves plenty of time for you to complete the registration process, which can take up to 6 months. It is common practice for employers to facilitate the registration and visa application processes. If this is not the case, once you have a job offer you should apply for a Temporary Skill Shortage visa (subclass 482). Other options include an Occupational Trainee visa and a Working Holiday visa.

The most common time for UK doctors to sample working in Australia is after FY2. The majority of roles available to these doctors are Resident Medical Officer (RMO) jobs. These may also be referred to as house officer jobs or hospital medical officer jobs and are the equivalent to junior clinical fellowships/Trust grade posts in the UK. Historically, the highest number of RMO jobs available is within A&E. For these roles, it may be a requirement for doctors to already have experience of A&E work in the UK. Beyond RMO jobs, there are specialty training positions that FY2 doctors can apply for. These may be called registrar jobs, trainee jobs, or senior house officer jobs. The majority of these positions will not accept overseas applicants, because full registration with the AHPRA is often a requirement. However, it may still be possible, at least further down the line.

17.4 New Zealand

Like Australia, New Zealand considers UK medical school training to be equivalent to its own. Therefore, UK medical school graduates do not have to sit additional examinations to work in New Zealand. UK medical school graduates are required to have a licence to practise medicine in the UK (gained by completing FY1) and must be of good standing with the GMC to be eligible to work in New Zealand. UK doctors can apply for a provisional licence, which allows them to work under the supervision of a senior medical practitioner. Typically, this provisional licence is converted to a full licence after 6 months, providing the supervisor raises no concerns. An application for a provisional licence will only be considered if the doctor has a confirmed job offer, with which supervision is provided. Doctors who have already completed some specialty training in the UK can apply for provisional vocational registration, to which the same rules apply.

There are many routes to job offers in New Zealand. UK doctors may wish to take part in the National Application Process, in which District Health Boards publish vacancies on their websites. Applications can be submitted via these websites, which can feel like an arduous task if submitting many of them. Jobs are also available via medical recruitment firms and locum agencies. In addition, it may be worthwhile contacting hospitals directly via their medical workforce department and providing a copy of your CV. In New Zealand, the training year for junior doctors commences in November/December. Jobs beginning in November/December are advertised around May and offers are usually made by August. Like in Australia, it is possible for UK doctors to start work in New Zealand in August. However, this is less common. Applications for jobs beginning in August should start around November. This leaves plenty of time for you to complete the registration process, which can take up to 6 months. It is common practice for employers to facilitate the registration and visa application processes. If this is not the case, once you have a job offer you should apply for an Essential Skills Visa or Holiday Working Visa.

Upon completion of FY2 in the UK, doctors are able to apply for house officer or junior registrar jobs in New Zealand. The work of a house officer in New Zealand is equivalent to the work of a foundation doctor in the UK. House officer jobs are great for gaining experience in certain specialties. However, they do not qualify as higher training. The work of a junior registrar in New Zealand is equivalent to the work of a core trainee in the UK. Junior registrar jobs are great for gaining experience in a specific specialty. Note that many of these positions require applicants to already have a minimum number of months experience in the specialty. These positions are also more contested than house officer ones.

17.5 Points to consider about working abroad

- **Doctors who have sampled working in a foreign healthcare system offer great value to the NHS and other UK employers.** This is because such doctors are able to use their overseas experience to influence and improve working styles in the UK. Working abroad is therefore commonly seen as an attractive feature to recruiters.

- **The most popular time for UK doctors to work overseas is after FY2. However, this is not the only opportunity to experience foreign healthcare systems** (even on a temporary basis). UK doctors in higher specialty training can also take time OOPT or OOPE (see *Chapter 13* for more detail).

- **Satisfying all of the requirements to work abroad is expensive.** *Table 17.1* outlines some of the notable costs associated with UK doctors working abroad.

Note: *Approximately £250 can be saved by relinquishing your GMC licence to practise medicine in the UK.*

17.5.1 Relinquishing your GMC licence to practise

Doctors who do not intend to practise medicine in the UK are able to maintain their GMC registration and relinquish their licence to practise. Those who opt for this pay a lower annual retention fee and are not required to revalidate. The GMC states that doctors who hold registration only must still act in accordance with Good Medical Practice guidance, remain subject to fitness to practise hearings and can be still be found on the UK medical register. When a doctor wishes to restore their licence, they will be asked to provide letters from their recent employers and regulators to prove good standing. Overall, this is a simple process.

WORKING ABROAD
CHAPTER 17

Table 17.1: Costs of working abroad

	Countries	Approximate cost
Examinations	USA: USMLE Parts I and II	£2000
	Canada: MCCQE Parts I and II	£3200
Registering with the relevant Medical Council/Authority	Australia	£1300
	New Zealand	£700
Criminal records check	All	£40
Notary public[1]	All	£150
Official visa medical[2]	All	£350
Temporary employment visa/permit	USA	£130
	Canada	£90
	Australia	£550
	New Zealand	£150
Medical indemnity insurance[3]	All	£80
Private medical insurance	All	Person-specific
Flights	All	£300 – £1000

[1] This is the process of verifying photocopies of signed documents. It is advised to get three copies of your documents.
[2] It is often a requirement to have a medical to work in foreign healthcare systems. There are only a few centres in the UK that are approved to perform this.
[3] It is easy to obtain a quote via your chosen UK indemnity insurance company website.

If a doctor decides to relinquish their GMC registration, things become more complicated. Granted, this will save you money on further retention fees. However, there have been cases in which doctors have encountered problems with re-registering when returning to work in the UK. For those who are working abroad on a temporary basis, it is generally advised to relinquish your GMC licence to practise medicine and maintain your GMC registration. For more information, see: ➔ **www.gmc-uk.org/registration-and-licensing/managing-your-registration/revalidation/revalidation-resources/revalidation-licence-to-practise-withdrawing-giving-up-restoring-appeals/licence-restoration**.

17.6 Top tips for medical students

- **If you are considering taking USMLE or MCCQE examinations, consider taking Part I around the same time as taking your medical finals.** The two curriculums will overlap and this way you will not have to relearn some of the key themes.

CHAPTER 18

Not having a career goal

Whilst at medical school and during your first few years of practising, it may seem like everyone around you knows what specialty they would like to pursue. This can be unsettling if you have not decided on your preferred career path. The best advice we can give is to keep your options open and not to worry. Try to build a CV that is not centred around one specialty, because this shows you are well rounded. Demonstrating commitment to a particular specialty should be the last piece of your puzzle. Be assured that working in different specialties throughout your FY1 and FY2 will make you more aware of your ideal career. Arranging a taster week in a specialty of interest can also play a big part. If at the end of FY2 you remain undecided about your career, a FY3 is a great option to explore different options, as is a FY4 and a FY5 if necessary. Asking for careers advice from doctors who are more senior than you can be incredibly valuable. They can provide first-hand knowledge of factors such as work–life balance, work-related stress, role variability, pay, job satisfaction and so on.

The scary reality of choosing a career in healthcare is that you may not have much experience in something before committing to it. It is therefore important to take an active approach in career planning. Ultimately, you will only be certain that you enjoy a particular career once you have tried it and there is always the option of applying for jobs in different specialties. A beneficial mindset to have is that if you are working in healthcare and gaining experience, you cannot take a backwards step. Flow diagrams like *Figure 18.1* are a lighthearted way to begin your search! Further resources that can help you decide which career path to take include:

- **BMA specialty explorer.** This is a tool for BMA members that supports your research into medical specialties. Users receive a personalised report of the top 10 medical specialties that match

THE ULTIMATE CAREER GUIDE FOR MEDICAL STUDENTS AND FOUNDATION DOCTORS

their answers: ➤ www.bma.org.uk/advice-and-support/career-progression/training/specialty-explorer.

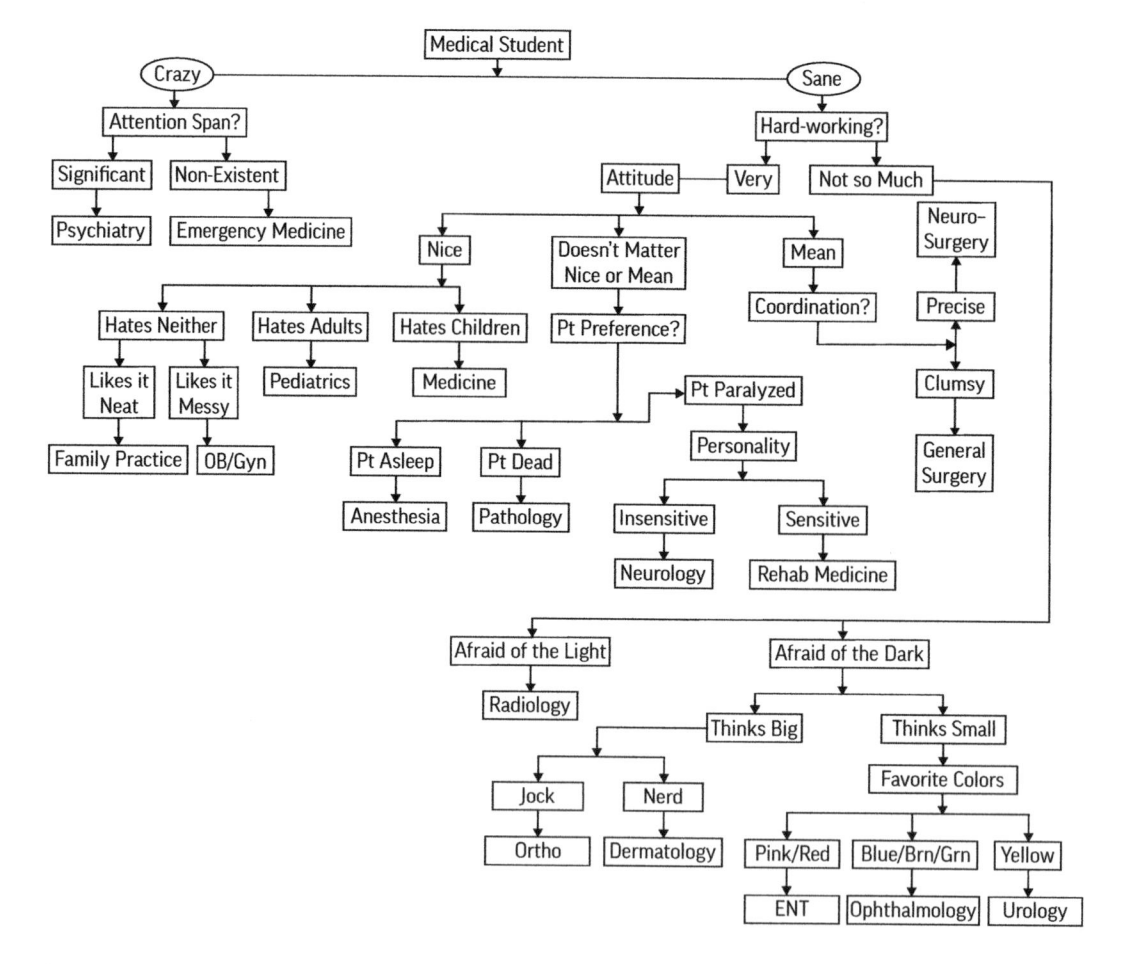

- **The London Professional Support Unit (Careers).** This resource offers individual, confidential and impartial careers support appointments with experienced career coaches and advisers. The unit also offers a Career Planning for Foundation Doctors E-Module, which follows the four-stage systematic, interactive and reflective SCAN Model (Self-awareness/Career exploration/Arriving at a Decision/ Next steps): ➤ https://london.hee.nhs.uk/careers-unit.

Figure 18.1: Specialty selection flow diagram.

Reproduced from ➤ www.medicalhumour.wordpress.com/2011/12/28/how-to-choose-medical-specialty-algorithm.

158

NOT HAVING A CAREER GOAL — CHAPTER 18

18.1 Top tips for medical students

- When you are on placement, a great question to ask consultants and senior registrars is – *if you were a medical student again, what specialty would you go into?* This question always triggers an interesting response because consultants and senior registrars often like to compare their careers with those of their friends in other specialties. Most importantly, it will also give you insight into the career satisfaction of senior doctors within different specialties.

18.2 Advice from the experts

Professor Chloe Orkin:

When did you first realise what specialty you wanted to pursue? And what were your reasons?
"I chose my specialty when my dear friend died of AIDS. I had always been interested in internal medicine and had been the prize student in virology and microbiology, so it was my destiny!"

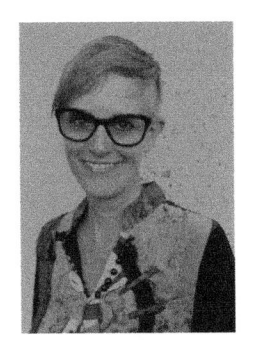

What advice can you give to those who do not know what their preferred specialty is and feel their CV might be lacking?
"Choose the specialty that fits who you want to be. Do you want to look after people with chronic conditions like HIV or MS? Do you want to work in a fast-paced environment like A&E? Are you a psychiatrist or are you a budding surgeon? What makes your heart race and who do you want to be (who are your role models) when you are doing your clinical work? This should give you a clue."

Dr Elaine Winkley:

When did you first realise what specialty you wanted to pursue? And what were your reasons?
"I did work experience at secondary school with an anaesthetist – it gave me a flavour – I followed that up with a Student Selected Module in 4th year at medical school. It was during this placement I developed relationships with individuals who are still role models and mentors. I selected an FY2 job in anaesthetics and sought opportunities in FY1 and FY2 to develop my portfolio and CV with anaesthetic-based projects and evidence."

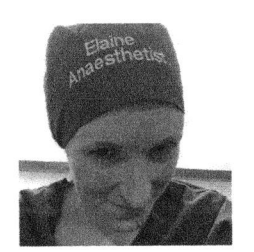

What advice can you give to those who do not know what their preferred specialty is and feel their CV might be lacking?

"Keep a broad base and be enthusiastic in every specialty even if you aren't sure – keep the doors open rather than slamming them shut. Do things you're passionate about – try to embrace every opportunity and keep a record of everything you do. It may seem tedious, but you need evidence to support any application."

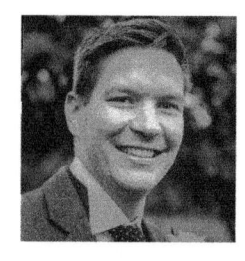

Mr Gareth Dobson:

When did you first realise what specialty you wanted to pursue? And what were your reasons?

"My undergraduate degree (BSc Neuroscience) and my medical school placements in neurosurgery and neurology confirmed neurosurgery as the specialty I wanted to pursue. Despite building my CV around neurosurgery when I applied after my FY3 year I was unsuccessful in obtaining an interview. I had ensured I had a 'plan B' in the way of a core surgical training application, from which I fortunately obtained an ENT-themed post. Again, the following year I applied for neurosurgical training, this time I was offered an interview, which did not go well. On the third time of applying, I finally managed to secure a post! Why neurosurgery? The complexity of the brain (an organ which not only controls what someone does but also who they are) and beauty of CNS anatomy was what initially interested me in neurosurgery. Experiencing the adrenaline rush when managing acute life-threatening cases, and the enjoyment of building such trust with patients to allow you to operate on their brain was what sold me on the specialty."

What advice can you give to those who do not know what their preferred specialty is and feel their CV might be lacking?

"Don't panic. Medicine has a vast range of specialties available and not everyone will know which one suits them. Commitment to specialty is only 'one box' on the application form, as long as you demonstrate that you are a well-rounded candidate, with a balanced CV then you should be OK. In my opinion simply having a genuine reason for pursuing a certain specialty is key."

NOT HAVING A CAREER GOAL   CHAPTER 18

Dr George Miller:

When did you first realise what specialty you wanted to pursue? And what were your reasons?
"I encountered Public Health Medicine for the first time during my foundation training, and immediately felt animated by the scope for influencing change on a wide scale."

What advice can you give to those who do not know what their preferred specialty is and feel their CV might be lacking?
"Even doing a little in each CV area will set you apart from much of the competition. Start immediately, and you will likely still have time to get ahead."

Dr Jeeves Wijesuriya:

When did you first realise what specialty you wanted to pursue? And what were your reasons?
"I suppose I knew I wanted to be a GP very early on in medical school. I really wanted a career that offered diversity and the opportunity to do lots of different things."

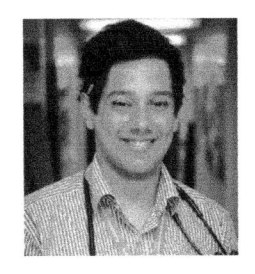

What advice can you give to those who do not know what their preferred specialty is and feel their CV might be lacking?
"I would say that it's never too late to get started. It is worth doing the things that really interest you, and to build relationships with people wherever you work. Try to find mentors or peers that will help advise and support you because that has been such an influential part of my career so far and has helped with the opportunities I have had. I know many people who didn't do much 'additional stuff' at medical school, and actually thrived afterwards by just asking what was available to them and looking for opportunities. I would encourage you to do the same!"

Dr Harrison Carter:

When did you first realise what specialty you wanted to pursue? And what were your reasons?
"I first got involved in basic science research looking at diabetic kidney disease in my BSc degree and fell in love with the kidney!

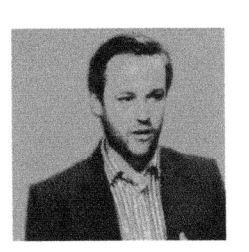

I then undertook some public health-related kidney research as part of my Public Health Master's at Cambridge before pursuing a quality improvement project as an Academic Foundation Doctor at Guy's Hospital. Renal medicine was the first specialty I took a 'deep dive' in and I never looked back!"

What advice can you give to those who do not know what their preferred specialty is and feel their CV might be lacking?

"Please don't worry. Focus on skills that you can translate across specialties. The fundamentals of being a good doctor are the same regardless of what you choose to do in the future. An inquiring mind and being intellectually curious is more important than anything else."

CHAPTER 19

Staying out of trouble

More than anyone, doctors are expected to act responsibly and be trustworthy. It is therefore crucial to keep a stain-free record for your behaviour when pursuing a successful career in medicine. Medical students who act inappropriately may be required to attend a fitness to practise meeting arranged by their medical school. At these meetings a panel will assess a medical student's fitness to practise. This assessment will determine if a medical student is able to continue their studies. Similarly, doctors who are accused of misconduct or malpractice will be subjected to a GMC investigation and fitness to practise hearing. The same is true for doctors who are given a criminal conviction or caution, and it is their legal obligation to declare it to the GMC and their employer. The GMC has the right to remove a doctor's licence to practise following a hearing if they believe it is necessary. If a doctor's licence remains intact after a hearing, the doctor will still be expected to provide an honest account of the hearing when applying for jobs. This may possibly hinder doctors' chances of securing competitive roles. Common pitfalls for medical students and doctors include:
- Posting inappropriate content on social media
- Disorderly conduct when drinking excess amounts of alcohol
- Inappropriate behaviour at society events or trips
- Use of recreational drugs.

Take extra care to not become involved in these activities. If you unfortunately find yourself in a situation where you are at risk of being subjected to a fitness to practise hearing, **you must seek professional help** from solicitors and organisations such as the BMA or your medical indemnity provider. These organisations have 24/7 helpline numbers that you can ring for confidential advice.
- BMA – Counselling and peer support for doctors and medical students: 0330 123 1245
- The MDU – medicolegal advice: 0800 716 646
- Medical Protection Society – medicolegal advice: 0800 561 9090